Rediscovering You

A 30 Day Self Care Guide for Modern Living

LADONNA NATURALE

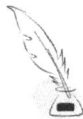

OTIS
PUBLISHING

First published by Otis Publishing 2024

Copyright © 2024 by LaDonna Naturale

First edition

This book was professionally typeset on Reedsy.
Find out more at reedsy.com

Introduction

In today's fast-paced world, stress has become a constant companion for many of us, silently weaving into the fabric of our daily lives. The relentless demands of modern living leave little room for quiet reflection or self-nourishment, leading to a widespread neglect of self-care. This oversight, seemingly inconsequential at first glance, can accumulate and manifest in ways that profoundly affect our physical, mental, and emotional health. Within this context, "Rediscovering You: A 30-Day Self-care Guide for Modern Living" emerges as a beacon of hope, offering insights and a practical pathway to weaving self-care into the very essence of our lives.

My vision for this book is clear and straightforward: to empower you with the understanding and tools necessary to transform your life through self-care. Recognizing that self-care is not a one-size-fits-all formula, I've tailored this guide to address the diverse needs and challenges adults and teens face. Whether you are navigating the complexities of adulthood or the turbulent years of adolescence, this book is your companion in the journey towards a more balanced and fulfilling lifestyle. What sets "Rediscovering You" apart is its structured yet flexible 30-day plan. Each day, you will be introduced to a new facet of self-care—a mindful exercise, a nutritional tweak, or a reflective practice—each explained with scientific insights, enriched with practical advice, and illuminated by personal reflections. These daily activities are designed to be accessible and actionable, making it easy to incorporate them into your routine, regardless of how busy you might be.

As someone who has navigated the choppy waters of stress and imbalance myself, I bring to this book a wealth of researched knowledge and a deep, personal understanding of the transformative power of self-care. My journey has taught me that wellness is both a science and an art, requiring knowledge, compassion, patience, and persistence.

In the following pages, you will explore self-care principles, practical daily activities, and advanced strategies for embedding these practices into your life for lasting well-being. But more than just a guide, this book is an invitation to step into a journey of self-discovery and self-compassion and rediscover your most authentic version.

Let me share a quote that has guided my journey: "Self-care is not a luxury; it is a necessity." This simple yet powerful statement captures the essence of our mission. As you turn each page, I encourage you to approach this journey with an open heart and a willing spirit, ready to embrace the small steps that lead to significant changes.

By the end of these 30 days, you will have a deeper understanding of self-care; you will have lived it, breathed it, and, most importantly, integrated it into your life. This is not just a promise of transformation; it is an assurance that with each step forward, you are not just rediscovering self-care; you are rediscovering you.

So, let us begin this journey together, knowing that every step we take is a step towards a more balanced, healthy, and fulfilled life. The path to rediscovering yourself starts now.

1

Chapter 1

The Self-Care Revolution

In the tapestry of human history, self-care has woven its presence subtly yet significantly, evolving alongside civilizations, cultures, and innovations. This chapter delves into the intricate evolution of self-care, unearthing its roots from basic survival practices to its current status as a holistic approach to wellness. It casts a light on the misconceptions shaped by modern marketing and expands the horizon of self-care beyond the physical to encompass mental and emotional health. Moreover, it celebrates the rich tapestry of global variations in self-care practices, advocating for a more inclusive understanding of what it means to care for oneself today.

The Evolution of Self-Care: Beyond Bubble Baths

Historical Perspective

Self-care is as ancient as humanity, rooted in the basic human instinct for survival. Early humans engaged in self-care practices not as a luxury but as a necessity for existence. These practices were rudimentary—seeking shelter, finding food, and tending to injuries. As civilizations advanced, so did the nuances of self-care. The ancient Egyptians indulged in baths and massages using aromatic oils, recognizing the importance of relaxation and physical well-being. In Ancient Greece, the philosophy of self-care was intertwined with the development of medicine, with Hippocrates proposing that diet, exercise, and rest were crucial to health. This historical journey underscores a significant shift: self-care evolved from survival tactics to encompass a broader spectrum of well-being, integrating physical health with spiritual and emotional wellness.

Modern Misconceptions

In contemporary society, the essence of self-care has been distorted, often marketed as a luxury or indulgence. This misrepresentation is a far cry from its foundational purpose. Self-commercializing self-care, emphasizing spa days, retail therapy, and beauty treatments, overlooks the core of caring for oneself. Such portrayals narrow the scope of self-care and alienate those who cannot afford these luxuries, perpetuating the myth that self-care is inaccessible to the average person. This misalignment with its historical roots highlights the need to recalibrate our understanding of self-care, steering it back to its inclusive and essential nature.

Broadening the Definition

To rectify modern misconceptions, broadening the definition of self-care is imperative. Proper self-care transcends the physical realm to encompass mental and emotional well-being.

It involves nurturing the mind with knowledge and reflection, caring for emotions through understanding and compassion, and fostering a connection with oneself and others. Such a comprehensive approach acknowledges that well-being is multidimensional, requiring attention and care in all aspects of life. This expanded definition not only aligns with the historical evolution of self-care but also makes it more accessible and relevant to everyone, regardless of their socioeconomic status.

Global Variations

The practice of self-care exhibits fascinating variations across different cultures, each adding a unique thread to the global tapestry of wellness. In Japan, the tradition of forest bathing, or shinrin-yoku, emphasizes the healing and rejuvenating power of being in nature. Scandinavian countries embrace the concept of hygge, finding comfort and joy in simple pleasures and warmth in the company of loved ones. In India, Ayurveda, an ancient system of medicine, advocates for a holistic approach to health, emphasizing the balance between mind, body, and spirit. These cultural practices highlight that self-care is not a monolithic concept but a diverse and rich collection of traditions and philosophies. Acknowledging and respecting these global variations enriches our understanding of self-care, reminding us of its universal relevance and the importance of viewing it holistically.

Reflective Exercise: Mapping Your Self-Care Journey

Take a moment to reflect on your self-care practices. How do they align with the historical evolution and broaden the definition of self-care? Do cultural traditions influence them, or have modern interpretations shaped them?

Consider your routine's balance between physical, mental, and emotional wellness. This reflective exercise serves as a starting point for reevaluating and enriching your approach to self-care, encouraging a holistic perspective encompassing all facets of well-being.

In summary, the evolution of self-care from a survival mechanism to a multifaceted approach to wellness underscores the dynamic nature of this practice. By challenging modern misconceptions and embracing a broader definition that includes mental and emotional health, we can reclaim the true essence of self-care. Furthermore, recognizing and celebrating the global variations in self-care practices enriches our understanding and connects us to the universal human experience of seeking health, happiness, and fulfillment.

Debunking Self-Care Myths: What It Is and Isn't

In the labyrinth of prevailing wellness discourse, self-care emerges as a sanctuary and a battleground, subject to myths and misconceptions that cloud its true essence. Far from being a mere trend or a commodity one can purchase, self-care is a foundational practice, elemental in its simplicity yet profound impact. This section aims to dismantle the myths surrounding self-care, laying bare its authentic nature and reinforcing its rightful place in personal health and wellness.

Myth vs. Reality

A pervasive myth portrays self-care as an act of selfishness, a notion steeped in misunderstanding. This belief stems from a skewed view of altruism, where caring for oneself supposedly detracts from one's ability to serve others.

Self-care is the wellspring from which our capacity to care for others flows. It replenishes our reserves of strength, compassion, and energy, preventing the all-too-common pitfalls of burnout and compassion fatigue. Another myth equates self-care with financial expenditure, conjuring images of lavish spa days and exotic retreats. While these can be part of one's self-care regime, they are not the entirety. Proper self-care often requires no financial cost, encompassing simple, everyday actions and decisions that honor our physical, mental, and emotional needs.

Not a One-Size-Fits-All

The diversity of human experience necessitates a self-care practice that is equally varied and personal. What soothes one person's stress might exacerbate another's, underscoring the importance of a tailored approach. For some, vigorous physical activity provides a release, while solitude and silence offer the greatest solace for others. This divergence in self-care practices is not a matter of right or wrong but of listening to and honoring one's needs and preferences. It invites an exploration of self, a trial and error process that, over time, reveals the unique constellation of practices that best serve one's well-being.

Beyond the Surface

The reduction of self-care to its physical aspects neglects the rich tapestry of mental and emotional well-being that it encompasses. Physical health, though visible and often measurable, is but one facet of a multidimensional construct. Cognitive and emotional self-care practices address the inner workings of the mind and heart—as crucial to overall health as the physical body. They include setting boundaries, engaging in therapy or counseling, practicing mindfulness and meditation, or simply allowing oneself to feel and express a full range of emotions. By expanding our understanding of self-care to include these aspects, we acknowledge the complexity of human health and the necessity of nurturing the mind and spirit alongside the body.

Self-Care vs. Escapism

In the quest for self-care, a fine line exists between genuine practices that foster health and well-being and those that serve as mere escapism. Often masquerading as self-care, the latter involves activities or behaviors to avoid facing uncomfortable emotions or realities. While escapism provides temporary relief, it ultimately sidesteps the root causes of distress, delaying true healing and growth. Genuine self-care, in contrast, involves confronting these challenges head-on, equipped with tools and practices that support healing and resilience. It requires courage to face what lies within, to sit with discomfort, and to seek growth and understanding through adversity.

In disentangling the myths from the reality of self-care, a more transparent, more accessible, and profoundly beneficial practice emerges. It is not a luxury indulgence but a fundamental aspect of living well. By embracing self-care in its fullness—acknowledging its necessity, diversity, depth, and distinction from escapism—we empower ourselves to lead lives marked by balance, health, and fulfillment.

The Science of Stress and the Role of Self-Care

Under the microscope of modern science, stress reveals itself not merely as an emotional response but as a complex physiological phenomenon deeply rooted in our evolutionary past. When faced with perceived threats, the human body activates its fight-or-flight response, a primal mechanism designed for survival. While beneficial in the short term, this response triggers a cascade of biochemical reactions: adrenaline floods the system, heart rate accelerates, muscles tense, and breathing quickens. Simultaneously, the brain's emotional centers are enlivened, sharpening senses and focus but, paradoxically, clouding judgment and rational thought. In the contemporary context, where threats are more psychological than physical, this once lifesaving response can become a source of chronic stress, leaving indelible marks on both body and mind.

In the labyrinth of modern life, where stressors abound, self-care emerges not as an indulgence but as a necessary countermeasure. This assertion is not merely anecdotal but is substantiated by a growing body of psychological and medical research. Studies reveal that self-care practices—from physical exercise and healthy eating to mindfulness meditation and adequate sleep—directly affect the stress response system. These activities mitigate the immediate physiological effects of stress and rewire the brain's neural pathways. Over time, individuals who engage in regular self-care demonstrate a heightened resilience to stress, characterized by a more subdued fight-or-flight response and an enhanced ability to return to equilibrium. The benefits of self-care, however, extend beyond the immediate horizon.

Chronic stress, left unchecked, is a formidable adversary, implicated in a host of long-term health issues, including cardiovascular disease, diabetes, depression, and a weakened immune system. By consistently integrating self-care into our daily routines, we offer ourselves a powerful shield against these potential afflictions. This protective effect is not merely physical. The psychological fortress it builds—bolstered by self-compassion, mindfulness, and emotional regulation—is a bulwark against the mental and emotional wear that chronic stress exacts over time.

In navigating the landscape of stress and self-care, it becomes critical to distinguish between the immediate relief provided by self-care activities and their cumulative health benefits. The allure of instant gratification, while understandable, often obscures the more profound value of sustained self-care practices. A single meditation session or a solitary nature walk offers a temporary respite from stress, lowering cortisol levels and calming the nervous system. Yet, the regular repetition of these activities, woven into the fabric of our daily lives, forges a durable defense against stress. This distinction is crucial, for it shifts the perception of self-care from a reactive measure—a band-aid applied in times of crisis—to a proactive strategy, a daily commitment to nurturing our well-being.

In this light, self-care transcends the realm of personal health, assuming a role of paramount importance in our collective well-being. As individuals fortified against the ravages of stress, we are better equipped to contribute positively to our communities, to offer support rather than succumb to despair, and to inspire resilience rather than spread discontent. Thus, in its most accurate form, self-care is an act of profound significance, a testament to our inherent capacity to adapt, heal, and thrive amidst the challenges of the modern world.

Customizing Your Self-Care: A Guide to Personalization

In the realm of self-care, the act of personal assessment stands as the cornerstone of a practice that is both nurturing and sustainable. This initial step, far from being a mere formality, requires a reflective gaze, a willingness to acknowledge one's current well-being across the physical, mental, and emotional spheres. It necessitates asking oneself probing questions: What aspects of my life are currently sources of stress? Which activities bring me joy and a sense of peace? How do I respond to solitude, to the company of others? The answers, though they might reveal vulnerabilities, are invaluable. They serve as the map that guides the customization of a self-care routine tailored to the individual's unique needs and aspirations.

With the blueprint of personal needs in hand, the next logical step is the integration of personal hobbies or interests into the self-care routine. This fusion is not merely about allocating time for leisure but about recognizing these activities as vital components of one's overall well-being. For some, this might mean the incorporation of creative pursuits such as painting or writing, activities that offer a reprieve from the mental clutter of everyday life, and an outlet for expression. For others, physical engagement—through yoga, hiking, or dance— provides a powerful antidote to stress, grounding the mind in the body and the present moment. This synergy between self-care and personal interests amplifies engagement and enjoyment and ensures that self-care feels less like a chore and more like a cherished part of one's daily routine.

Adapting self-care practices to fit various lifestyles, schedules, and resource availability is equally critical. In a world where time is often scarce, self-care can evoke feelings of guilt or frustration, particularly among those juggling multiple responsibilities. The solution lies not in the wholesale adoption of time-consuming practices but in the artful integration of self-care into the crevices of daily life. It might manifest as a brief meditation during the morning commute, a mindful walk during lunch, or the practice of gratitude in the moments before sleep. For those with erratic schedules or limited resources, it emphasizes the importance of flexibility and creativity in pursuing well-being, encouraging online resources, free community programs, or simply the healing power of nature. Lastly, the acknowledgment that one's needs and circumstances are in constant flux underpins the approach to self-care as a dynamic, evolving practice. In its relentless unpredictability, life brings about anticipated, unforeseen changes that can significantly impact one's well-being. It is here that the practice of periodic reassessment becomes crucial. This reflective and honest process allows for the recalibration of self-care practices in response to life's shifts. It recognizes that a practice that once served as a source of solace might lose its resonance, just as new challenges might necessitate new strategies for care. This fluidity, far from being a sign of inconsistency, is a testament to the individual's commitment to self-awareness and growth, to the recognition that self-care, at its core, is about nurturing oneself through the ebb and flow of life.

In navigating these steps—personal assessment, the integration of interests, adaptation to lifestyle, and the acknowledgment of evolving needs—the individual crafts a self-care practice that is not only personalized but deeply embedded in the fabric of their daily existence. This approach, marked by introspection, flexibility, and a commitment to growth, ensures that self-care remains a vital, nourishing presence in one's life, capable of adapting to the ever-changing landscape of human experience.

The Impact of Self-Care on Relationships

In the intricate web of human connections, the self-care thread weaves a pattern of resilience and strength, fortifying the individual and the bonds that tether them to others. At the heart of this dynamic, the relationship with oneself acts as the fulcrum around which all other relationships orbit. When nurtured through self-care, this central relationship blooms, its petals unfurling to touch and enrich the myriad connections that make up the tapestry of one's social world. The act of caring for oneself, therefore, transcends the boundaries of the individual, casting ripples across the waters of interpersonal relationships.

The significance of self-care in enhancing personal relationships is multifaceted. At its most fundamental, it fosters a sense of self-worth and confidence, qualities that radiate outward, coloring interactions with a hue of positivity and openness. A person grounded in self-care approaches relationships, not from a place of neediness or dependency but from a position of fullness and abundance. This shift in perspective transforms the nature of interactions, making them sources of mutual growth and enrichment rather than battlegrounds for validation and approval. Moreover, the self-care journey often involves introspection and self-discovery, processes that unearth the authentic self. When one operates from this core of authenticity, relationships gain depth and meaning, founded on genuine connection rather than superficial exchange. Modeling self-care is crucial in the social environment, serving as a silent teacher of wellness and balance. This is particularly potent in the context of family and close relationships, where habits and attitudes observed in one member often ripple through to others. When parents prioritize self-care, they implicitly teach their children the value of wellness, setting the foundation for a lifetime of healthy habits. Friends observing the transformative effects of self-care in a peer may find themselves inspired to embark on their wellness paths. Thus, the individual act of self-care becomes a collective movement, gradually shifting the culture of communities towards one that values and prioritizes well-being.

At the intersection of self-care and relationships lies the crucial concept of boundaries. Self-care involves recognizing and respecting one's limits, needs, and desires—a recognition that naturally extends to establishing healthy boundaries in relationships. These boundaries, far from erecting barriers between individuals, serve as the framework within which healthy interactions flourish. They allow for the expression of needs and the negotiation of space, fostering a climate of respect and mutual understanding. Moreover, clarity with well-defined boundaries simplifies communication, reducing potential conflict and misunderstanding. In this way, self-care is the architect of a relationship landscape marked by openness, respect, and reciprocal care.

One of the most profound impacts of self-care on relationships is the enhancement of empathy and understanding. The journey of self-care is, at its core, an exercise in compassion— compassion towards oneself. This inward-directed compassion, once cultivated, does not remain confined to the self. It expands outward, informing interactions with others. A person attuned to their own needs and emotions develops a heightened sensitivity to the needs and feelings of others. This empathetic stance transforms relationships, making them conduits for deep, meaningful connections. Conversations grounded in empathy open doors to understanding, allowing individuals to transcend their perspectives and truly see the world through another's eyes. In conflicts, empathy acts as a bridge, facilitating resolution and healing.

Moreover, self-care equips individuals with the tools to manage their emotional states, reducing the likelihood of projecting personal frustrations and insecurities onto others. This emotional regulation benefits the individual and stabilizes their interactions with others, providing a steady foundation for relationships to grow and thrive. Through the lens of empathy, the challenges and struggles of others are met with kindness and support rather than judgment or dismissal. This supportive stance, rooted in genuine understanding and care, strengthens the bonds between individuals, weaving a fabric of relationships resilient to the trials of life.

In the realm of personal connections, self-care emerges not as an isolated act but as a vital component of social wellness. Its influence permeates the layers of individual relationships, transforming them from within. Self-care acts as a catalyst for positive change through the enhancement of personal relationships, the modeling of healthy habits, the establishment of effective communication and boundaries, and the cultivation of empathy. It redefines how individuals relate to themselves and each other, fostering a society that values wellness, balance, and mutual respect.

Defining Your Self-Care Needs: A Reflective Exercise

Self-reflection, in its quiet power, acts as the compass by which we navigate the often tumultuous seas of our inner worlds. It invites us to pause, to turn inwards, and to listen —truly listen— to the whispers and roars of our deepest needs and desires. This process, far from a mere exercise in introspection, is the foundation upon which personal self-care is constructed. It demands honesty, openness, and a willingness to confront our luminous strengths and shadowed vulnerabilities.

To initiate this reflective exercise, a series of questions serve as the lanterns lighting the path to self-discovery. These inquiries probe the dimensions of our lives that often elude conscious consideration yet hold sway over our well-being. "What moments in my day do I look forward to, and what do I dread?" This question alone can unveil patterns of joy and discomfort, guiding us to activities that nourish our souls. "When do I feel most at peace with myself? Conversely, when do I feel dissonance or discord within?" Such questions peel back the layers of our daily existence, revealing the textures of our emotional landscapes. "How do my surroundings influence my mental and emotional state?" prompts an examination of the interplay between environment and well-being, pushing us to consider changes that might foster a more nurturing space.

With the revelations unearthed through these inquiries in hand, the task becomes prioritization. This stage acknowledges a fundamental truth: our resources—time, energy, or material— are finite. Thus, not every need can be met with equal immediacy or intensity. Prioritization demands that we weigh the urgency and importance of our needs, distinguishing between what must be addressed and what can wait. For some, this might mean focusing on alleviating physical pain or discomfort, recognizing that without a stable foundation of physical health, psychological and emotional well-being remain elusive goals. For others, mending strained relationships or addressing mental health struggles may take precedence.

The act of setting goals emerges naturally from the process of prioritization. In this context, goals are not lofty aspirations or distant dreams but achievable targets, stepping stones toward enhanced well-being. Practical goals share certain characteristics; they are specific, lending clarity to the desired outcome; they are measurable, allowing for the tracking of progress; they are achievable, grounded in realism rather than fantasy; they are relevant, aligned with our deepest needs and values; and they are time-bound, endowed with a sense of urgency and a deadline for accomplishment.

Setting a goal to incorporate a ten-minute meditation into each morning, for example, meets these criteria. It is specific in its action, measurable by its daily completion, achievable within the constraints of most schedules, relevant to the need for mental clarity and emotional calm, and time-bound to the start of each day. Another goal might be to engage in physical activity three times a week, a commitment that, while modest, holds the potential for profound impacts on physical and mental health. These goals, rooted in the self-knowledge gleaned through reflection, become the milestones marking our progress on the self-care journey.

This reflective exercise is not a one-time endeavor but a cyclical spiral that deepens with each iteration. As we evolve, so too do our needs and desires, demanding that we return to the well of self-reflection, reassess our priorities, and adjust our goals accordingly. This adaptive approach ensures that our self-care practices remain attuned to the ever-changing rhythms of our lives, resonating with our current realities rather than echoing past needs. It is through this ongoing dialogue with ourselves that we cultivate a self-care practice that is not static but dynamic, not burdensome but liberating, and not imposed but chosen —a practice that, in its depth and authenticity, becomes a wellspring of strength and serenity in the flux of life.

The Intersection of Self-Care and Productivity

In the realm where self-care meets productivity, a prevailing myth casts a long shadow, suggesting that dedicating time to oneself is stolen from work, creativity, and the relentless pursuit of success. This notion, deeply ingrained in the fabric of hustle culture, fails to recognize the symbiotic relationship between caring for oneself and achieving peak performance. Far from being a zero-sum game, where the investment in one's well-being comes at the expense of productivity, self-care emerges as the foundation for sustainable productivity.

Research, cutting through the fog of misconceptions, illuminates the truth about this relationship. Studies in psychology and neuroscience reveal that self-care practices — from physical exercise to mindfulness meditation — have tangible effects on the brain. These activities stimulate the production of neurochemicals such as dopamine and serotonin, enhancing mood and motivation. Furthermore, they foster neuroplasticity, the brain's ability to form new neural connections, improving cognitive functions such as memory, attention, and creativity. In this light, self-care is not a detour from the path to productivity but a conduit, fostering an environment within which the mind can flourish.

The concept of mental rest, often overlooked in productivity discussions, warrants a closer examination. In a culture that glorifies constant activity and the relentless pursuit of goals, the notion of rest is frequently dismissed as unnecessary, even indulgent. Yet, cognitive science tells a different story. Mental rest, achieved through self-care practices such as short breaks during work or study, meditation, or leisure activities, is crucial for cognitive function. It allows the brain to consolidate memories, integrate new information, and solve complex problems more effectively. This rest period acts as a reset button, clearing the mental clutter accumulating with prolonged focus, enhancing clarity, decision-making, and creativity.

Practical strategies for integrating self-care into daily routines offer a road map for navigating the intersection of well-being and productivity. One such strategy involves deliberately scheduling short self-care breaks throughout the workday. These breaks, ranging from a five-minute walk to a brief meditation session, provide the mind with the respite to maintain focus and creativity over long periods. Another approach is setting clear boundaries around work hours and ensuring dedicated time for rest and leisure activities, safeguarding against burnout and fostering long-term productivity.

Adopting a mindset that views self-care as an integral part of a productive life is crucial. This shift in perspective, recognizing that caring for oneself and achieving one's goals are not mutually exclusive but mutually reinforcing, paves the way for a more balanced, fulfilling approach to work and life. It challenges the deeply held belief that success is the product of relentless effort alone, inviting a more nuanced understanding that recognizes the role of well-being in sustaining high-performance levels.

Overcoming Barriers to Self-Care: Time and Guilt

Two formidable obstacles often stand in the way of self-care: the scarcity of time and the weight of guilt. Though seemingly impossible, these barriers can be navigated with introspection, practical strategies, and a shift in perspective.

Identifying Barriers

The first step in overcoming these obstacles is to recognize their presence and understand their origins. The perception of not having enough time for self-care is often rooted in pri- oritizing external demands—work, family, social obligations— above one's well-being. This skewed hierarchy of priorities is not a reflection of selfishness but a manifestation of soci- etal pressures that valorize busyness and productivity at the expense of health and happiness. Similarly, guilt arises from a misalignment of values, where caring for oneself is mistakenly viewed as indulgent or selfish, a misconception propagated by the same societal norms that glorify sacrifice and martyrdom for others' sake.

Strategies to Overcome Guilt

A reevaluation of its role in overall well-being is essential to dismantle the guilt associated with self-care. This process begins with acknowledging that self-care is not merely a personal indulgence but a critical component of health and functionality. It enables individuals to recharge, to foster resilience, and to maintain the capacity to support and care for others. Recognizing this broader impact of self-care helps reframe it as an act of responsibility rather than selfishness. Further, engaging in dialogue with oneself and others about these feelings of guilt can illuminate their irrational nature and foster a supportive environment for the practice of self-care. Sharing experiences and struggles with self-care can also help normalize these practices and counteract the stigma surrounding them.

Time Management for Self-Care

The challenge of integrating self-care into a busy schedule necessitates a strategic approach to time management. This strategy begins with an audit of one's daily activities, identifying periods consumed by non-essential tasks or inefficiencies. Even in the most packed schedules, pockets of time often go unnoticed or underutilized—moments that could be reclaimed for self-care. The key lies in planning and allocating specific times for self-care activities, just as one would for work meetings or family commitments. This deliberate scheduling ensures that self-care is woven into the fabric of daily life rather than relegated to the margins. Moreover, adopting flexible self-care practices that can be adapted to varying time constraints— such as short meditation sessions, brief outdoor walks, or even mindful breathing exercises during commutes—can make self-care more accessible amidst the hustle of daily routines.

Incorporating self-care into daily life also involves setting realistic expectations about the duration and type of self-care activities. Dispelling the notion that self-care requires large blocks of time or elaborate setups can free individuals to embrace more simple, spontaneous forms of self-care.

This might include a five-minute journaling session, a brief stretch during a break at work, or a few moments of gratitude reflection before bedtime. These small, manageable practices accumulate over time, contributing significantly to one's well- being without necessitating substantial time commitments.

Reframing Mindsets

At the core of overcoming barriers to self-care lies the need for a profound shift in mindset. This shift moves from perceiving self-care as a luxury or an optional add-on to life to recognizing it as a foundational element of health and well-being. Such a reorientation involves challenging deeply ingrained beliefs about productivity, worthiness, and self-sacrifice, questioning the societal narratives that equate constant busyness with success and self-neglect with virtue.

Embracing self-care as a non-negotiable aspect of life requires a conscious effort to redefine success and worth, acknowledging that actual achievement encompasses professional or social milestones and maintaining one's health, happiness, and inner peace. This redefinition broadens the scope of what is valued and celebrated in life, placing well-being at the center.

Additionally, cultivating a compassionate attitude towards oneself is crucial in this mindset shift. Self-compassion involves treating oneself with the same kindness, understanding, and forgiveness that one would offer to a friend in distress. It allows for moments of rest, self-care practices, and the pursuit of joy without the shadow of guilt or the pressure of unrealistic expectations. By fostering self-compassion, individuals can navigate the challenges of integrating self-care into their lives with grace and resilience, viewing setbacks not as failures but as opportunities for growth and reaffirming their commitment to well-being.

As individuals embark on this journey of reframing their mindsets, they unlock the potential to transform their relation- ship with self-care. This transformation is not a destination but an ongoing process, a continuous dialogue between one's evolving needs and the practices that nurture and sustain them. Through this dialogue, self-care becomes not an obstacle to overcome but a path to traverse, a journey marked by discovery, healing, and the profound realization that caring for oneself is
the most fundamental act of living fully.

Self-Care for Different Life Stages

The fabric of self-care is woven with threads of varying thickness and color, each representing the different stages of life. From the vibrant hues of adolescence to the softer tones of older age, the needs and practices of self-care evolve, reflecting the changing landscapes of physical, mental, and emotional well-being. This evolution is not linear but cyclical, with each stage bringing unique challenges and growth opportunities.

In adolescence, the surge of hormonal changes and the quest for identity cast a complex backdrop for self-care. During these formative years, practices that foster self-esteem and body positivity are crucial. Engaging in sports or physical activities can be a powerful conduit for channeling energy and emotions while laying the foundation for a healthy lifestyle. Equally important are mental health practices, such as journaling or engaging in open conversations with trusted adults, which provide a safe space for navigating the tumultuous waters of teenage emotions. Peer support groups also play a pivotal role, offering a sense of belonging and a buffer against the isolation that can accompany the adolescent search for self.

Transitioning into young adulthood, self-care takes on new dimensions as individuals face the pressures of career building, relationships, and, for many, the responsibilities of parenthood. Time management becomes critical, balancing personal well- being with professional and familial duties. Mindfulness and stress-reduction techniques, such as deep breathing exercises or short meditative practices, can be woven into the fabric of daily life, providing islands of calm amid chaos. Nutrition and training are pillars of physical self-care, emphasizing sustainable practices that fit busy schedules. Additionally, fostering solid social connections during this stage enriches emotional well-being and establishes a support network for navigating life's challenges.

Self-care practices often shift towards maintenance and prevention as individuals progress into mid-life. Health screenings have become more relevant, serving as a proactive approach to well-being. This stage may also prompt a reevaluation of life goals and aspirations, leading to a deeper exploration of hobbies and interests that bring joy and fulfillment beyond professional achievements. The onset of physical changes necessitates a more focused approach to physical activity, emphasizing flexibility, strength training, and cardiovascular health. Mindfulness and reflective practices gain depth, encouraging a reconnection with one's core values and reassessing life's priorities.

Advancing into older age, the emphasis of self-care shifts towards preserving independence and enhancing quality of life. Physical activity, tailored to individual capability, remains a cornerstone, with activities such as walking, swimming, or yoga contributing to mobility and balance. Nutrition is essential, focusing on foods that support cognitive function and overall health. Social engagement becomes vital to emotional well- being, combatting the isolation accompanying this life stage. Through classes, hobbies, or volunteering, lifelong learning keeps the mind active and engaged, fostering a sense of purpose and connection.

The concept of inter-generational self-care introduces a rich tapestry of shared experiences and wisdom, bridging the gap between ages. This practice acknowledges that self-care is not confined to individual silos but is a collective endeavor enriched by the contributions of each generation. For instance, grandparents teaching grandchildren the art of gardening imparts knowledge and offers physical activity, connection to nature, and nutritional benefits. Similarly, younger family members can introduce older relatives to technology, opening new avenues for learning and social connection. Shared physical activities, such as family hikes or yoga sessions, provide opportunities for bonding while promoting health across generations.

These shared practices underscore the universality of self-care and its relevance across the lifespan. They remind us that, regardless of age, caring for oneself and others is a thread that connects us, weaving a more robust, more resilient fabric of
community and well-being.

The Role of Community in Self-Care

In the intricate dance of individuality and collectivism, the notion of self-care often finds itself mislabeled as a solitary exercise, a misconception that overlooks the profound impact of community.

While personal in its texture, the fabric of our well-being is interwoven with the threads of social connections and communal support. These ties, extending beyond the confines of our immediate surroundings, offer strength, inspiration, and a shared sense of purpose, reinforcing the scaffolding upon which our self-care practices rest.

Community Support

The significance of a supportive community in bolstering self-care cannot be overstated. Humans, inherently social beings, thrive on connection and the affirmation of belonging. The presence of a compassionate community provides a mirror reflecting our struggles and triumphs, normalizing the challenges of self-care while celebrating its successes. This reciprocal exchange of support and encouragement acts as a catalyst, sustaining motivation and amplifying the impact of self-care practices. Within such circles, wisdom is shared, strategies are diversified, and realizing that one is not alone in their quest for well-being becomes a source of comfort and resilience.

Finding Your Tribe

Finding or cultivating a community aligned with one's self-care values and interests might seem daunting. Yet, the seeds for such connections often lie dormant within our existing networks, awaiting the right conditions to germinate. Initiating conversations about self-care with friends, family, or colleagues can uncover shared interests and values, laying the groundwork for deeper, more meaningful connections. For those seeking new tribes, local clubs or groups centered around activities such as yoga, hiking, or meditation offer fertile ground for planting the roots of the community. These physical and symbolic spaces become sanctuaries where like-minded individuals converge, drawn together by a shared commitment to well-being.

Group Self-Care Activities

The collective pursuit of self-care within these tribes manifests in a myriad of group activities, each designed to foster belonging while enhancing collective well-being. Group meditation sessions, for instance, harness the power of shared energy, creating a profound sense of connection and tranquility. Similarly, community gardening projects promote physical activity and connection to nature and cultivate a shared understanding of responsibility and achievement. These activities, while diverse in their execution, share a common thread: the belief that well-being flourishes in the soil of community, nurtured by the hands of collective effort and care.

Digital Communities

In an era where digital landscapes often mirror, and at times eclipse, the physical realms of interaction, the role of online platforms in fostering self-care communities has surged to the forefront. Social media, forums, and dedicated apps offer expansive, borderless spaces where individuals from varied backgrounds and geographies converge around shared interests in self-care. These digital tribes, while lacking in physical presence, provide a wealth of resources, support, and inspiration, accessible with but a click. Here, stories and strategies are exchanged, transcending geographical limitations and weaving a global tapestry of self-care. Yet, this digital communion has its challenges. The anonymity and scale of online interactions can sometimes dilute the essence of community, rendering it impersonal. Navigating this digital domain requires discernment. One must seek spaces that prioritize authenticity, respect, and genuine connection over mere numbers and surface-level engagement.

In the confluence of community and self-care, we find a dynamic interplay between the individual and the collective, a dance of give-and-take that enriches both. The community acts as a mirror, a sounding board, and a cheering squad, reflecting our efforts, amplifying our successes, and cushioning our stumbles. It reminds us that while the path of self-care is personal, it need not be lonely. The journey, shared with others, becomes less about reaching a destination and more about the connections forged along the way, the collective strides towards well-being, and the realization that every individual bloom in

the garden of self-care adds beauty to the whole.

Crafting Your Self-Care Mission Statement

In self-care, a personal mission statement serves as a lighthouse, casting a steady, illuminating glow over the waters of daily life, guiding the way through calm and tumultuous seas. This beacon, rooted in one's deepest values and loftiest goals, offers clarity amidst the fog of day-to-day decisions, ensuring that each choice and action aligns with the overarching vision for well-being.

The essence of a self-care mission statement lies in its ability to distill complex aspirations into an explicit, potent declaration. It is a manifesto declaring one's commitment to nurturing the self, advocating for personal needs, and honoring the intrinsic value of health and happiness. The benefits of articulating such a statement are manifold. It acts as a constant reminder of one's priorities, especially in moments when external demands threaten to overshadow personal well-being. It fosters a sense of purpose, lending meaning to routine self-care practices by linking them to broader life goals. Most importantly, it serves as a compass, orienting one's daily choices towards the true north of holistic well-being.

The crafting of this statement begins with introspection, a deep dive into the reservoir of one's values, beliefs, and aspirations. What principles guide your life? What visions of well-being do you hold dear? The answers to these questions form the foundation for your statement. Reflect on the aspects of self-care that resonate most deeply with you; these range from physical health and mental clarity to emotional resilience and spiritual fulfillment. Consider, too, your aspirations—how you wish to feel, the qualities you aspire to embody, and the impact you desire to have on your life and those around you.

Armed with this insight, the next step is to distill these elements into a coherent, concise statement. This is not an exercise in verbosity but in precision, carving out an aspirational and actionable declaration. The statement should encapsulate what self-care means to you, weaving together your values, goals, and the practices that bring them to life. It might read, "My mission is to honor my body and mind by engaging in practices that foster strength, serenity, and self-compassion, guiding me toward a life of fulfillment and purpose." Though it may require time and reflection, this process culminates a powerful articulation of your self-care ethos.

Living your self-care mission statement is where its true power unfolds. It becomes the lens through which daily choices are viewed, the criteria by which actions are judged. This document breathes life into a routine, transforming boring tasks into meaningful steps toward a larger goal. It calls for mindfulness, a conscious engagement with each moment, ensuring that even the most straightforward decisions—what to eat, how to spend free time, and when to rest—align with your mission. In practice, this might mean choosing nourishing foods that honor your body, carving out time for activities that replenish your spirit, and setting boundaries that protect your time and energy. In these daily acts, guided by your mission statement, the grand vision for well-being is realized, one choice at a time.

Yet, as constant as the north star, change is an inherent aspect of life. Just as the seas shift and the winds change direction, so too do our needs and circumstances evolve. This fluidity demands that our self-care mission statement, while steadfast in its core values, remains adaptable. Revisiting and revising this statement becomes integral to the self-care practice, reflecting growth and change. Periodically, take stock of where you are on your self-care journey, assessing how your needs have shifted and your practices have adapted. This might occur at natural transition points—such as the start of a new year, a birthday, or a significant life change—but can also be prompted by a sense that your current practices no longer align with your deepest needs.

In this revisiting, ask yourself: Does my mission statement still reflect my values and goals? Have new priorities emerged that necessitate a shift in focus? The answers to these questions guide the revision process, ensuring your statement remains relevant and resonant. This could mean refining your focus, emphasizing mental health more, or incorporating aspects of social well-being. Or it might involve a broader reimagining of your self-care vision, adapting to new understandings of yourself and your place in the world.

The self-care mission statement is not a static document but a living, breathing part of your journey. It evolves as you evolve, reflecting your growth, learning, and aspirations. It is both a declaration of intent and a map, guiding your daily choices and illuminating the path toward holistic well-being. Through crafting, living, and revising your statement, you engage in a profound dialogue with yourself, a conversation that deepens your commitment to self-care and enriches your journey toward a life of health, happiness, and fulfillment.

The Importance of Boundary Setting in Self-Care

In the tapestry of self-care, boundaries emerge as threads that define and protect the space where our well-being can flourish. These invisible lines, both firm and permeable, delineate the extent of our domain, safeguarding our physical, emotional, and mental landscapes from the encroachments of external demands and expectations. Boundaries, in their essence, are declarations of self-respect and self-preservation, signaling to ourselves and others the value we place on our health and happiness.

To grasp the significance of boundaries in self-care, one must first understand their nature and purpose. Boundaries are not barriers erected in isolation or defiance but rather parameters facilitating healthy interactions and personal growth. They enable us to engage with the world from a place of strength and autonomy, choosing how we expend our energy, with whom we share our time, and to what extent we open ourselves to the influences of our surroundings. By asserting our boundaries, we honor our needs, preferences, and limits, creating a safe space for self-care practices to take root and thrive.

Identifying where boundaries are needed or could be strengthened requires a reflective and honest assessment of our current state of well-being. This process involves tuning in to our physical and emotional responses to various aspects of our lives—work, relationships, social commitments—and listening for signs of discomfort, resentment, or fatigue that may indicate a crossed boundary. Perhaps the chronic overextension at work leaves no time for rest or the habitual acquiescence to social obligations that drain rather than fulfill. Recognizing these areas of discontent is the first step toward reclaiming our space and energy for self-care.

Once areas needing stronger boundaries have been identified, setting and communicating these boundaries effectively is the challenge. While daunting, this endeavor is rooted in clear, assertive communication that respects our needs and those of others. It begins with clarity about what we are willing to accept and where we draw the line, articulated directly yet compassionately. For instance, setting a boundary around work hours may involve a conversation with colleagues or superiors about not responding to emails after a specific time, framing this limit not as a refusal to engage but as a measure to ensure quality and focus during working hours. Similarly, communicating boundaries in personal relationships might mean expressing the need for solitude or declining invitations that conflict with self-care practices, doing so in a way that conveys love and respect for both oneself and the relationship. However, setting boundaries is only half the equation; respecting these boundaries completes the circle of self-care. This respect begins with honoring our boundaries and resisting the urge to bend them for fear of disappointment or conflict. It requires a steadfast commitment to our well-being, trusting that the short-term discomfort of asserting our boundaries pales to the long-term benefits of a life that aligns with our needs and values. Equally important is respect for the limits set by others and recognition of their right to self-care and autonomy. This mutual respect fosters relationships built on understanding and support, where self-care is not a solitary endeavor but a shared value.

Boundaries emerge as essential choreography in the intricate dance between individual well-being and the web of social interactions. They allow us to move through the world with grace and intention, engaging fully and openly yet constantly from a place of self-awareness and self-respect. Through the thoughtful setting and honoring of boundaries, we cultivate a life that nurtures our well-being and enriches our interactions with others, proving that self-care, in its most accurate form, is both a personal and collective good.

2

Chapter 2

Morning Alchemy: Transforming Beginnings

With its gentle nudge toward consciousness, the first light of dawn offers not just the start of a new day but a canvas for transformation. This pristine moment, untainted by the residue of yesterday's concerns or the weight of today's obligations, holds the potential for a deliberate creation of experience. It whispers a powerful question: How will you sculpt the hours to come?

Morning Rituals to Start Your Day Right

Establishing a Routine

The rhythm of the morning sets the tempo for the day. A consistent morning routine is the spine of one's daily architecture, providing structure and stability. Like the unwavering path of the sun across the sky, a set sequence of actions reassures the mind, signaling that, despite the world's unpredictability, some things remain under our control. It's about crafting a personal liturgy that sanctifies the start of each day, transforming ordinary moments into a sacred sequence that primes the body and mind for the possibilities ahead.

Mindful Awakening

Consider the first conscious breath of the day as an anchor, grounding you in the present. Practices such as gentle stretching awaken the body softly, respecting its need to ease from the vulnerability of sleep into the vitality required for wakefulness. Similarly, gratitude journaling, even if it's just listing three things you're grateful for, shifts the mind's lens from scarcity to abundance, coloring the day with a hue of positivity. This mindful awakening recalibrates our internal narrative, choosing hope and gratitude as the day's foundational themes.

Hydration and Nutrition

The body, after a night's rest, craves replenishment. A glass of water, perhaps with a squeeze of lemon, rehydrates and kick-starts the digestive system, symbolizing the cleansing of yesterday and the preparation for today's nourishment. Following this, a breakfast that balances macronutrients fuels both body and mind, laying down the energy reserves necessary for the day's demands. Imagine your body as a garden; hydration is the morning dew, and a nutritious breakfast, the sunlight and soil nurturing growth.

Visualization and Goal Setting

With the body awakened and nourished, the mind turns to the abstract landscapes of thought and imagination. Visualization, the act of painting the day's desires and objectives in the mind's eye, serves as a rehearsal, priming the psyche for the roles and scenes ahead. Following this visualization with goal setting, where aspirations are distilled into tangible actions, ensures that the day's script aligns with the broader narrative of one's life. Setting achievable goals each morning is akin to plotting way points on a map, guiding the day's journey with intention and purpose.

In a world where mornings often succumb to the tyranny of the urgent, crafting a beginning that serves as an alchemy of productivity and peace is a radical act. It's about choosing to greet the day not as a series of tasks to be endured but as a landscape to be cultivated with care. Each morning, then, becomes not just a repetition of routines but a ritual of transformation, turning the lead of the mundane into the gold of the meaningful.

Mindful Commuting: Transforming Transit into Self-Care

Redefining Commute Time

The daily commute, often perceived as a mere interlude between the personal sanctuary of home and the demands of the workplace, holds untapped potential for self-care. Rather than a void of lost time, this transition can be reimagined as a fertile period for nurturing the mind and spirit. It is an invitation to reclaim these moments, transforming them into a sanctuary of calm and a practice ground for mindfulness amidst the bustle of transit. By shifting our perspective, we uncover the opportunity to infuse these intervals with intention, making every journey a stepping stone toward tranquility and preparedness for the day ahead.

Mindful Breathing Exercises

Breathing, the most fundamental of our body's rhythms, offers a bridge to mindfulness that can be crossed in any setting, including commuting. Mindful breathing exercises, focused on the deliberate inhalation and exhalation of breath, anchor us in the present, clearing the mental clutter that accumulates with anticipation of the day's challenges or the residues of yesterday's trials. This practice can be seamlessly integrated into any commute, serving as a tool to dissolve stress and foster a state of centered calm. By concentrating on the breath, we engage the parasympathetic nervous system, diffusing the stress response and cultivating an oasis of peace amidst the transit chaos.

Audio books and Podcasts

The enrichment of the mind, often relegated to the margins of our packed schedules, finds a perfect venue in the time spent commuting. Audio books and podcasts, spanning a wealth of topics from philosophy to personal development, transform transit time into a mobile classroom or seminar. This auditory consumption of knowledge and insights elevates the mind and redefines the commute as a period of intellectual and emotional growth. The careful selection of uplifting and educational content inspires, motivates, and prepares the listener for the day ahead, turning what was once idle time into a productive and enriching experience.

Observational Mindfulness

Observational mindfulness during commuting involves a conscious engagement with our immediate environment, turning our attention outward to absorb the details of the world around us. This practice, rooted in the principles of mindfulness, encourages a non-judgmental awareness of the present moment. By observing the interplay of light and shadow, the diversity of people and their interactions, or the dance of nature and urban landscapes, we cultivate a sense of connection to the world beyond our concerns. This connection fosters a feeling of belonging and perspective, reminding us of our place within the larger tapestry of life. Observational mindfulness serves as a practice of presence and a celebration of the world's complexity and beauty, often overlooked in the rush of daily routines.

Commuting transforms from a mere transition to an opportunity for self-care, and we discover the power of perspective and intention. By reclaiming these moments for mindfulness, learning, and observation, we enrich our daily existence, turning every journey into a pathway toward personal growth and peace.

Workplace Wellness: Self-Care for the Busy Professional

Desk Ergonomics

In the realm where productivity intersects with self-preservation, the physical arrangement of our workspace emerges as a silent yet potent influencer of well-being. Ergonomics, the science dedicated to designing and arranging items people use so that the people and things interact most efficiently and safely, offers a beacon of guidance. For the professional tethered to their desk, ergonomics translates into cultivating space that minimizes strain and promotes physical ease. Begin with the chair, the throne of the working domain; it should support the spine's natural curve, with feet resting firmly on the ground or a footrest. The monitor, that window to the digital world, must be positioned at eye level, a comfortable arm's length away, to avoid the slump toward the screen that burdens the neck and shoulders. The keyboard and mouse, tools of the trade, should allow the wrists to rest in a neutral position, avoiding the arch that invites discomfort. Though subtle in its adjustments, this orchestration of workspace elements sings a melody of comfort and efficiency, turning the hours spent at the desk into a symphony of productivity free from the discord of physical discomfort.

Micro-breaks

Time, that relentless march forward, often becomes a tyrant in the office, dictating long stretches of uninterrupted labor. Yet, within its iron grip lies the potential for rebellion, small acts of liberation known as micro-breaks. These brief pauses in the workday, spanning mere minutes, are oases of restorative calm. They invite the eyes to wander from the screen's glow, basking instead in the distance or the soft, natural light spilling through a nearby window. The mind also finds respite, momentarily stepping away from the task to bask in a snippet of meditation or savor the simple act of sipping water. Even the body, long held in the static embrace of sitting, unfurls through stretching, reconnecting with the often-forgotten joy of movement. These micro-breaks, sprinkled like way points throughout the day, serve as reminders that productivity flourishes not in relentless exertion but in the balance between effort and ease.

Healthy Snacking

Amidst the ebb and flow of deadlines and meetings, nourishment often becomes an afterthought, a need muted by the multitude of tasks demanding attention. Yet, the sustenance we provide our bodies shapes the energy and focus we bring to these tasks. Healthy snacking, the art of choosing foods that fuel rather than deplete, becomes a pillar of workplace wellness. Imagine snacks as small, nutrient-dense gifts to oneself, packages of energy that sustain and invigorate. A handful of almonds, rich in healthy fats and protein, offers a steady release of energy, while a crisp apple delivers a natural sweetness packed with fiber and hydration. Even drinking water, that most basic form of nourishment, becomes a ritual of refreshment, clearing the mind and replenishing the body. By elevating snacking from a mindless habit to a mindful practice, we ensure that our fuel sources are as refined and purposeful as the work we aspire to produce.

Boundary Setting

In the tapestry of professional life, boundaries act as the threads that delineate personal space, demarcating where work ends and personal life begins. The modern professional, often besieged by the blurring of these lines, finds sanctuary in the deliberate setting of boundaries. It starts with the temporal, the establishment of work hours beyond which the tools of labor are laid to rest. This temporal boundary, a fortress against the encroachment of professional demands into the sanctity of personal time, requires vigilance and discipline to maintain. Communication, too, must be tempered by boundaries, with the expectation set that responses will flow within designated hours, preserving the tranquility necessary for rest and rejuvenation. With its tendrils extending into every corner of life, the digital realm demands its own set of boundaries, a conscious choice to disconnect, to step away from the constant ping of notifications and the glow of screens. In setting these boundaries, we carve out space for life beyond work, a domain where self-care is not just possible but prioritized, ensuring that a well-nourished, well-rested self fuels our professional endeavors.

In the workplace crucible, wellness emerges not as a static achievement but as a dynamic practice woven through the choices we make and the boundaries we set. It's a testament to the belief that our work, while a vital part of our identity and purpose, flourishes most when balanced with the care we invest in ourselves.

Mindfulness Practices for Stress Reduction

Introduction to Mindfulness

In the vast expanse of human experience, moments teem with the potential for mindfulness. This practice beckons us to dwell fully in the present, attentive to the nuances of our existence. Mindfulness, an ancient tradition now validated by modern psychology, invites an intimate engagement with the here and now, a deliberate attention that filters out the cacophony of past regrets and future anxieties. This practice, rooted in the simple act of noticing, cultivates a space where the mind can repose in its natural calm, untethered from the narratives that often besiege it. The benefits, far-reaching and transformative, encompass a diminution of stress, an enhancement of focus, and an amplification of gratitude, weaving a tapestry of well-being that enriches the fabric of daily life.

Breathing Techniques

Amidst the whirlwind of daily obligations, breathing

emerges not merely as an involuntary function but as a sanctuary of tranquility, a haven accessible in even the most tumultuous of times. Various breathing techniques, each a unique alchemy of rhythm and focus, offer pathways to centering and serenity. The 4-7-8 method, inhaling deeply for four counts, holding the breath for seven, and exhaling smoothly for eight, serves as a balm, slowing the heartbeat and inviting the nervous system to rest. Another technique, diaphragmatic breathing, emphasizes the full engagement of the lungs, drawing air deep into the belly, a practice that signals safety to the brain, diffusing the tendrils of stress. When practiced with intention, these methods act as anchors, grounding us amid life's storms and reminding us of the power held in a single breath.

Mindful Walking

Walking, often perceived as a means to an end, holds within it the seeds of mindfulness, transforming each step into an opportunity for connection with the present. Mindful walking, a practice that marries the rhythm of steps with the cadence of breath, invites a deep engagement with the environment. It beckons the senses to awaken, to observe the intricacies of the landscape, the play of light on leaves, the symphony of sounds, from the rustle of grass to the murmur of distant voices. This walking meditation, even if woven into the fabric of a few brief minutes, bridges the gap between body and mind, external world, and internal landscape, fostering a sense of peace and groundedness in the simple act of moving through space.

Body Scan Meditation

Within the confines of our flesh and bones lies a universe, a complex system of sensations and emotions often overlooked in the rush of daily living.

The body scan meditation, a deliberate journey through this inner cosmos, invites a focused awareness that begins at the crown and gently sweeps down to the toes. This exploration, guided by a gentle curiosity, uncovers pockets of tension where stress has lodged, manifesting as tightness or discomfort. As awareness caresses these spots, a conscious release unfolds, an unclenching that allows relaxation to seep into the furrows of strain. This practice, organized and compassionate, not only fosters a release of physical tension but also cultivates a profound connection with the body, recognizing it as a barometer for stress and a vessel for well-being.

In mindfulness, each breath, step, and moment of focused attention counterbalance the pressures that besiege us, a recalibration of our relationship with time and existence. These practices, breathing techniques, mindful walking, and body scan meditation are not mere activities but invitations to a way of being that honors the present as the ultimate repository of life's richness. Through mindfulness, we navigate the currents of daily life not as passive vessels but as active participants, attuned to the depth and breadth of our experiences, enriched by paying attention.

The Art of Saying No: Protecting Your Energy

Recognizing Energy Drainers

In the tapestry of daily life, threads of various hues represent the myriad requests and commitments vying for our attention and energy. Amidst this colorful array, darker and more insistent strands symbolize the demands that deplete our vitality and cloud our clarity. Identifying these energy drainers necessitates a vigilant awareness of our internal landscape, an attunement to the subtle shifts in our emotional and physical states that signal depletion. This discernment is cultivated through reflection, a conscious examination of how specific engagements affect our sense of well-being. Does the thought of a particular commitment evoke a sense of dread or exhaustion? Do specific interactions leave us feeling drained rather than enriched? Though simple, these questions serve as a compass, guiding us toward recognizing activities and obligations that sap our strength, allowing us to navigate our energies more judiciously.

Assertiveness Training

The art of assertiveness lies at the heart of saying no, a skill that, once honed, empowers us to communicate our refusals with confidence and clarity. Assertiveness training begins with acknowledging our inherent right to prioritize our needs and set boundaries. It involves cultivating a language of self-assurance that communicates refusal without apology or excessive explanation. Key to this practice is using "I" statements, expressions that root our refusals in our feelings and needs rather than external judgments or criticisms. "I feel overwhelmed by my current commitments and need to focus on my well-being" offers a declaration of self-care, framing the refusal as a personal necessity rather than outright rejection. This approach not only softens the impact of the refusal on the recipient but also reinforces our agency over our time and energy.

Prioritizing Self-Care

At the intersection of self-awareness and assertiveness lies the crucial act of prioritizing self-care, a deliberate choice to place our well-being at the forefront of our decisions. This prioritization demands a reevaluation of the societal narratives that equate busyness with worth and self-neglect with virtue. It calls for a recalibration of values, recognizing that productivity and fulfillment stem from a wellspring of vitality and peace, not from the relentless pursuit of external validation. Practically, this means permitting ourselves to decline invitations or obligations that conflict with our self-care practices, viewing these practices not as optional luxuries but as non-negotiable elements of our daily lives. In this space of prioritization, we find the freedom to cultivate a life that resonates with our deepest needs and aspirations, a life where saying no becomes an affirmation of self-respect and self-love.

Practical Scenarios

Navigating the practical scenarios that demand our refusal is akin to walking a tightrope, a balance between honoring our needs and maintaining harmony in our relationships. Consider the common situation of an overextended calendar, where the addition of another commitment threatens to tip the scales from busy to unmanageable. A script for refusal, in this instance, might read, "I appreciate your invitation and would love to contribute under different circumstances. However, I'm currently at capacity with commitments and must honor my need for rest and balance." This respectful and sincere response communicates the refusal clearly while leaving the door open for future engagement.

Another frequent scenario involves requests for assistance that, though well-intentioned, infringe upon our limited time and energy reserves. An assertive refusal might be,

"Helping you with this project sounds like a wonderful opportunity, but I'm prioritizing some personal commitments and self-care practices now. I'm unable to take on additional responsibilities." This refusal, while firm, acknowledges the value of the request and the difficulty of the decision, fostering understanding and respect.

In these scenarios and countless others like them, the scripts we employ to serve as templates, customizable to the nuances of each situation but always rooted in the principles of assertiveness, respect, and self-care. They remind us that saying no is not an act of rejection but a declaration of our commitment to our well-being, values, and priorities. Through practice, the art of saying no becomes less daunting, transforming into a tool that safeguards our energy, nurtures our vitality and enriches the quality of our engagements. In this artistry, we find the strength to protect our space and power and the grace to navigate our relationships with integrity and compassion.

Digital Detox: Balancing Technology Use

In an age where the digital realm infiltrates every crevice of our daily existence, a digital detox emerges not as a luxury but as a necessity, an antidote to the constant barrage of notifications, emails, and social media scrolling. This section navigates the waters of our digital consumption, urging a recalibration of our relationship with technology, transforming it from a master to a tool that serves rather than diminishes our quality of life.

Assessing Digital Use

The initial step towards a balanced digital life begins with a candid assessment of our current engagement with technology.

This introspection involves tracking the hours spent in the glow of screens, acknowledging the habitual reach for the phone upon waking, and compulsively checking emails throughout the day. The objective here is not self-reprimand but awareness, illuminating patterns of use that veer towards excess. By quantifying our digital consumption, we lay bare its impact on our well-being, noting how each hour online detracts from sleep, in-person relationships, and immersion in the tangible world around us. This awareness becomes the bedrock upon which we build our strategies for detoxification, a map guiding us away from digital saturation towards a more harmonious existence.

Setting Digital Boundaries

With a clear understanding of our digital habits, the following stride involves the establishment of boundaries, delineat- ing when, where, and how technology infiltrates our lives. Designating screen-free times, perhaps the first hour upon waking and the last hour before sleep, carve out sacred spaces for presence and reflection, untainted by the digital world's demands. Similarly, declaring certain home areas, such as the bedroom or dining table, as sanctuaries accessible from screens fosters environments conducive to relaxation and genuine connection with loved ones. While simple in concept, these boundaries demand discipline in practice, a commitment to uphold the sanctity of our designated screen-free zones and
times, and pushing back against digital intrusion.

Mindful Technology Use

The crux of a digital detox lies not in the wholesale renunciation of technology but in its mindful use, a conscious engagement that elevates our human experience rather than detracting from it. This mindfulness involves intentionality in our interactions with digital devices, asking ourselves whether each action—opening an app or responding to a notification— aligns with our broader goals and values. It invites a pause before the reflexive reach for the phone, a moment to question whether this engagement serves a purpose or merely fills a void. In this space of mindfulness, technology becomes a tool wielded with precision, enhancing productivity, learning, and connection, rather than a vortex that saps time and attention.

Alternative Activities

The vacuum left by reduced screen time beckons to be filled, not with the longing for what was relinquished but with activities that nourish the body, mind, and spirit. This transition is an invitation to rediscover hobbies and passions sidelined in the digital age, activities that engage the senses and spark joy. Delving into the pages of a book, brush in hand against canvas, or fingers dancing over piano keys, we reconnect with the tactile pleasures of the physical world. Outdoor pursuits, from a stroll in the park to an exhilarating hike through the wilderness, rekindle our bond with nature, grounding us in the beauty and serenity of the natural world. Even the simple act of cooking a meal from scratch or tending to a garden becomes a meditation, a celebration of the tangible and the transient. In these alternative activities, we find a respite from the digital and a deeper connection to the essence of living, a richness that screens can never replicate.

The steps outlined in this section guide us in the delicate dance with technology toward a rhythm that resonates with our inherent need for connection, creativity, and calm.

Through assessment, boundary setting, mindful engagement, and embracing alternative activities, we craft a relationship with the digital world that enhances rather than traps, a balance that allows us to harness the benefits of technology without becoming tethered to its demands. This recalibration is not a retreat from the modern world but a reclamation of our autonomy. It is a declaration that in the vast expanse of human experience, the most vibrant hues are found not on screens but in the unfiltered panorama of life itself.

Nutritional Self-Care: Eating for Wellness

In the intricate dance of sustenance and vitality, the alchemy of nutrients ignites a cascade of reactions; each bite is a spell cast upon our holistic health. The threads that bind the fabric of our mental, physical, and emotional well-being are dyed in the hues of the foods we consume, painting a picture of health that is as vibrant as it is varied. This connection, undeniable in its influence, beckons a mindful approach to nourishment, an invitation to treat each meal as a sacred communion between the body and the earth's bounty.

The direct link between nutrition and our holistic health operates not merely on the physiological plane but extends its roots deep into the emotional and cognitive soils of our being. Foods rich in nutrients work in concert to fortify the body's defenses, enhance cognitive capabilities, and stabilize emotional landscapes. Omega-3 fatty acids, abundant in walnuts and flaxseeds, weave a tapestry of neural connections, improving memory and warding off the fog that often clouds our thoughts. Simultaneously, the vibrant array of antioxidants in berries and leafy greens scours the body for free radicals, purging the physical form of potential harm. At the same time, the humble mineral magnesium, nestled within dark chocolate and avocados, acts as a balm for frayed nerves, soothing anxiety with its gentle touch.

Amidst the rush of modern life, eating often becomes a task to be checked off a list, a mechanical refueling devoid of presence or pleasure. Yet, mindful eating practices beckon us to slow this hurried pace, to savor not just the flavors but the very act of nourishment itself. This practice invites a full sensory engagement with our meals. This attentiveness enhances the experience and fosters a deeper connection with our body's hunger signals and satiety. It teaches us to recognize the difference between physical hunger and emotional voids masquerading as cravings, guiding us to choices that satisfy the palate and the body's needs. Through this attentiveness, we learn to honor our hunger, to approach each meal with gratitude rather than guilt, and to find joy in the simplicity of a ripe, sun-warmed tomato or the earthy richness of a mushroom.

Crafting balanced, nutritious meals becomes an act of self-care, a deliberate choice to nourish the body with what it needs to thrive. The principles of balance and variety guide this culinary journey, ensuring that each plate becomes a mosaic of macronutrients and micronutrients. The harmony of proteins, fats, and carbohydrates, in proportions that cater to the body's nuanced needs, fuels our activities and repairs our tissues. Proteins, the building blocks of cells, lend their strength to muscles and bones, while carbohydrates, the body's preferred energy source, ignite the fires of activity and thought. Fats, long vilified yet essential, envelop cells in a protective embrace, facilitating the absorption of fat-soluble vitamins that guard against disease. When played against a varied diet, this nutritional symphony ensures that no nutrient is left unexplored, offering the body the full spectrum of health-promoting compounds.

Hydration, often overshadowed by the focus on food, emerges as a cornerstone of nutritional self-care. Water, the most primal of needs, courses through our veins, carrying life to every cell, whispering of vitality and purity. It lubricates joints, nourishes the brain, and purges the body of toxins, acting as the medium through which the symphony of life unfolds. Drinking water, rhythmic and routine, becomes a ritual of renewal, a momentary return to the simplicity of being. In its clarity, we find a reflection of our need for purity and replenishment, a reminder that sometimes, the simplest acts can be the most profound.

In nutritional self-care, we find not just a strategy for health but a philosophy of living, a recognition that each choice we make at the table reflects our reverence for the life within us. It is a practice that bridges the gap between the body and the mind, between sustenance and the soul, inviting us to approach each meal with intention, gratitude, and a deep understanding of the nourishment it offers. Through this practice, we learn to eat and feed ourselves in the truest sense, honoring the body's wisdom and the earth's generosity with every mindful bite.

The Power of Movement: Exercise as Self-Care

Benefits Beyond Physical Health

In the intricate ballet of existence, movement orchestrates a symphony within, echoing far beyond the confines of physical well-being into the vast chambers of mental and emotional states. This alchemy, where each stride, stretch, and sway transmutes inertia into vitality, reveals exercise as a catalyst for an enriched life. Engaging in regular physical activity initiates a cascade of biochemical reactions— endorphins surge, stress hormones wane, and the mind, once a storm of thoughts, finds its calm in the eye of the storm. This equilibrium, born of movement, fosters a resilience that armors the psyche against the slings and arrows of daily stressors, painting a portrait of well-being as complex as it is complete. Here, in the sweat and pulse of exertion, we uncover a sanctuary for the soul, a space where the world's tumult fades into the background, leaving only the rhythm of breath and the heart's beat.

Finding Joy in Movement

Amidst the myriad modalities of exercise, the quest for joy in movement beckons as a siren song, luring us to explore the waters of physical activity until we find the stream that quickens our pulse with exertion and exhilaration. This journey, marked not by the monotony of obligation but by the thrill of discovery, invites us to sample the spectrum of movement—from the graceful arcs of yoga to the exhilarating rush of cycling, the steady cadence of jogging to the playful buoyancy of swimming. Each form of exercise, a world unto itself, offers a unique blend of challenges and rewards, beckoning us to listen to our bodies' whispers and hearts' desires. In this exploration, we find the key to sustainability in exercise—a joyous engagement that beckons us back, day after day, not out of duty but out of desire.

Integrating Movement into Daily Life

The canvas of our daily lives, often segmented into blocks of work, rest, and recreation, holds within its structure the potential for a seamless integration of movement. This endeavor, far from requiring the upheaval of our routine, calls for a creative reimagining of the mundane—a choice to take the stairs rather than the elevator, a decision to bike to work instead of driving, or the simple act of standing rather than sitting during a phone call. These activity threads, woven into the fabric of our day, form a tapestry of movement that enriches our existence without demanding time we believe we don't have. Even household chores, from gardening to cleaning, emerge as opportunities for physical engagement, transforming the ordinary into the extraordinary. In these moments, movement becomes not an addition to our day but a redefinition of it, a shift in perspective that reveals the potential for exercise in every action.

Setting Realistic Goals

Setting goals, those beacons that guide us toward well-being, demands a delicate balance between aspiration and attainability. In physical activity, this balance hinges on understanding our current capacities and the gentle stretching of our limits. Goals, articulated with clarity and grounded in reality, serve as milestones on the self-care journey through exercise. They are not lofty peaks that loom intimidatingly on the horizon but stepping stones that mark the progress of our endeavor. While modest, a goal as simple as a daily ten-minute walk lays the foundation for a habit of movement, a small victory in the more extensive health campaign. Gradually, these goals evolve, expanding in ambition as our strength and stamina grow, yet permanently anchored in the principle of achievable challenge. This approach, measured and mindful, ensures that exercise remains a source of joy and empowerment, a wellspring of vitality rather than a well of frustration.

In this landscape of movement, where the body becomes both the instrument and the expression of care, each step, each stretch, and each breath becomes a testament to the power of physical engagement to transform not just our physique but our psyche. It is a reminder that in moving, we engage in a dialogue with our deepest selves, a conversation that spans the languages of muscle and mind, heart, and soul. Through this dialogue, we discover not just the strength of our limbs but the resilience of our spirit and our heart's capacity to embrace joy in the simple act of living fully, vibrantly, in the world of motion.

Nature as Therapy: Outdoor Activities for Well-being

Scientific Benefits of Nature

Within the embrace of the natural world, a quiet revolution unfolds, one that recalibrates the soul and the synapses with equal finesse. Empirical research, a steadfast ally in the quest for understanding, casts a revealing light on this symbiosis between humanity and the earth. It elucidates the mechanisms by which the mere act of immersing oneself in nature acts as a balm for the psyche and a tonic for the brain. The verdant hues of forests and the expansive blue of skies and waters instigate a reduction in stress markers, a softening of the heart's rhythms, and a quieting of the mind's constant chatter. Further scrutiny reveals enhancements in mood, a buoyancy borne of the earth's unscripted beauty and the unhurried pace of life it exemplifies. Cognitive functions, too, bask in nature's glow, with attention and memory finding rejuvenation amidst the simplicity of natural landscapes. This confluence of benefits, a testament to nature's healing prowess, invites a deliberate integration of outdoor activities into the fabric of daily life, weaving together humans and habitats that enrich both.

Ideas for Outdoor Activities

The spectrum of activities that beckon under the open sky is as vast and varied as the landscapes that inspire them. For those whose spirits soar with exertion, the rhythmic cadence of a hike through undulating trails offers physical engagement and communion with the earth beneath their feet. Cycling, with the wind as a companion, transforms the act of movement into a journey; each pedal strokes a narrative of discovery and delight. For souls drawn to the reflective calm of the water, kayaking on a serene lake or the gentle discipline of fishing provides a meditative interaction with the liquid element. Even the simple act of gardening, hands deep in the soil, becomes a dialogue with life itself, nurturing growth that mirrors the internal cultivation of well-being. These activities, selected not for their novelty but for the resonance they find within the heart, serve as conduits to the therapeutic essence of nature, each a thread in the tapestry of outdoor well-being.

Urban Nature

The quest for nature's solace need not lead to remote wilderness; even within the concrete embrace of urban landscapes, pockets of green and blue persist, whispering of tranquility amidst the tumult. Parks, those oases of greenery, beckon with their promise of respite and recreation, a space where trees and lawns offer a backdrop for leisure and activity. Rooftop gardens, a testament to human ingenuity, elevate the act of cultivation to the skies, turning barren expanses into verdant plots that soothe the eye and the spirit. Even walking, when directed along tree-lined streets or towards local water bodies, becomes an exploration of the urban wild, a discovery of nature's persistence. For those ensconced in cityscapes, these ventures into urban nature serve as vital reminders of the earth's enduring presence, a call to seek and celebrate the natural enclaves that survive amid the asphalt.

Seasonal Considerations

The wheel of the year turns, bringing with it a kaleidoscope of climates and colors, each season a unique backdrop for engagement with the outdoors. In the burgeoning life of spring, nature invites exploration, its trails adorned with the tender hues of new growth and skies echoing the calls of returning birds. Activities such as bird watching or the simple pleasure of a walk amidst blooming flora celebrate the season's vibrancy and align the internal rhythms with the renewal cycle. With its abundance of light and warmth, summer opens the doors to water-based activities, from swimming in the cool embrace of lakes to the leisurely exploration of coastlines. The mellow richness of autumn calls for hikes through forests aflame with color, a sensory feast that preludes the reflective quiet of winter. Even in the cold embrace of the latter season, nature beckons with the crisp clarity of air and the silent beauty of snow-covered landscapes, inviting activities that revel in the serene austerity, from snowshoeing to the simple act of building a snowman. This attunement to the seasons, a dance with the earth's rhythms, ensures a year-round connection with the outdoors, a sustained engagement that nourishes the body and the spirit in equal measure.

In this exploration of nature as therapy, the invitation

stands open to weave the natural world into the essence of our being, allowing its rhythms to guide our own, its beauty to inform our vision, and its vastness to expand our hearts. Through deliberate engagement with outdoor activities tailored to personal inclinations and the unique tapestry of the seasons, we find an enhancement of well-being and a deepening of our connection to the earth. In this connection, we discover the essence of well-being, a harmony between self and surroundings that elevates our life experience to a more prosperous, vibrant hue.

Creative Outlets for Emotional Expression

Identifying Creative Interests

In the tapestry of self-care, creative expression emerges as a vibrant thread, weaving through the fabric of daily existence with the potential to transform mundane moments into instances of profound discovery. This process begins with exploring creative outlets that resonate with individual interests and emotional landscapes. The spectrum of creativity spans far-reaching domains—from the rhythmic strokes of a paintbrush to the structured cadence of poetry, from the tactile manipulation of clay to the digital creation of images. Each medium offers a unique pathway to self-expression, an invitation to articulate the inarticulable, to give form to the formless emotions that dwell within. To unearth these interests, one must listen attentively to the inner voice that whispers inclinations and curiosities, guiding the hands and heart towards the medium that best mirrors the soul's language.

Therapeutic Benefits of Creativity

In its myriad forms, the act of creation serves not merely as an endeavor of artistic pursuit but as a conduit for emotional catharsis and psychological resilience. Engaging in creative activities initiates a dialogue with the self. This non-verbal communication transcends the limitations of language, offering a sanctuary for emotions to be felt, examined, and transformed. This inherently therapeutic process harnesses the power of creativity to navigate the complexities of the human psyche, providing a means to process and release emotions that might otherwise remain trapped in the recesses of the mind. The rhythmic repetition of stitches in knitting, the focused attention required in sculpting, and the immersive flow state induced by painting —all these acts of creativity act as meditations, reducing stress and invoking a sense of calm. Moreover, bringing something new into existence fosters a sense of accomplishment and self-efficacy, counteracting the feelings of helplessness that often accompany emotional turmoil.

Starting Small

The journey into creative expression need not begin with grand projects or ambitious undertakings; instead, it flourishes in cultivating small, manageable endeavors that invite regular engagement. Incorporating creativity into one's routine can start with as simple an act as doodling in the margins of a notebook, crafting a haiku before bedtime, or experimenting with recipes in the kitchen. These small acts of creation, easily woven into the fabric of daily life, serve as stepping stones, gradually building confidence and skill. They remind us that creativity is not the exclusive domain of the artistically trained but a universal language, accessible and understandable to all who seek its solace.

Creating Without Judgment

At the heart of creative exploration lies the imperative to detach from the inner critic, that voice that whispers doubts and magnifies flaws, casting shadows on the joy of creation. To create without judgment is to approach each creative endeavor with a mindset of exploration and enjoyment, valuing the process over the product. This perspective encourages experimentation, allowing for missteps and imperfections as integral elements of the creative journey. It fosters an environment where the act of creation becomes a source of joy rather than anxiety, where the focus remains on the act of making and the emotional release it provides rather than on the critique of the outcome. In this space, free from self-criticism and perfectionism, creativity blossoms, unfettered and pure, a true reflection of the self in its most authentic form.

In exploring creative outlets for emotional expression, we find not just a method for stress reduction or a means to process emotions but a celebration of the human capacity to create and transform inner turmoil into external beauty. It is a reminder that within each of us lies an artist, a creator capable of manifesting our inner worlds into tangible forms, offering solace to the self and a gift of understanding and connection to the world beyond.

Nighttime Routines for Better Sleep

Importance of Sleep

In the sanctuary of the night, sleep beckons as the ultimate restorer, weaving its restorative threads through the fabric of our being, mending the wear of day's exertions. This nightly renewal transcends physical recuperation, embedding itself in mental clarity and emotional equilibrium.

The science of sleep elucidates its pivotal role in memory consolidation, forti- fying the immune system, and regulating mood, underscoring sleep not as a passive state but as an active, vital process of rebalancing and healing. The architecture of sleep, with its cycles of REM and non-REM stages, constructs the foundation upon which our daytime consciousness depends, influencing our capacity for learning, creativity, and emotional resilience. Thus, cultivating practices that enhance sleep quality becomes a keystone habit, a foundational ritual that supports the edifice of overall health and well-being.

Developing a Soothing Routine

As twilight deepens, the initiation of a soothing pre-sleep rou- tine serves as an invitation to unwind, signaling the impending descent into repose to the psyche. This sequence, a personal litany of calm, might unfurl through the gentle stretching of limbs, releasing the physical knots of the day's labors. The embrace of warm, herbal teas, their steam-carrying whispers of relaxation, further soothe the senses, preparing the palate for rest. Reading, where words become the lullaby for the mind or the soft, musical strains of calming music, can usher in tranquility, easing the transition from wakefulness to sleep. This routine, repeated with the devotion of ritual, becomes a stepping stone on the path to restful nights, a series of stepping stones leading gently to the shores of sleep.

Sleep Environment

In sleep, the environment reigns as sovereign, its elements conspiring to either welcome rest or ward it away. The dominion of light, with its power to sway the circadian rhythms that govern our sleep-wake cycles, demands careful negotiation. The banishment of blue light, emitted with insidious intensity by screens, becomes imperative as night falls, preserving the sanctity of natural sleep signals. The embrace of darkness, facilitated by blackout curtains or sleep masks, cocoons the sleeper in velvety shadows conducive to slumber. Temperature, too, plays its part in this orchestration, with cooler air mimicking the body's natural nocturnal dip in warmth, nestling us into a deeper sleep. And amidst the din of urban existence, the cultivation of silence or the gentle hum of white noise buffers the intrusion of the world's clamor, cradling the sleeper in an auditory womb of peace.

Dealing with Sleep Challenges

Yet, for many, the voyage to sleep's embrace is fraught with challenges, with nights spent navigating the turbulent waters of insomnia or the fitful unrest of disturbed sleep. In these moments, the arsenal of relaxation techniques becomes invaluable, offering tools to dismantle the barriers to rest. The practice of progressive muscle relaxation, where tension is consciously tensed and then released, traverses the body's landscape, softening the soil of stress that impedes sleep. Guided imagery, a mental excursion to realms of peace and serenity, diverts the mind from the whirlpool of anxious thoughts, anchoring it in the calm of imagined tranquility. For minds that churn with the unresolved residue of the day, journaling offers a release, a transference of worries from psyche to page, clearing the mental decks for sleep's arrival. Wielded with patience and persistence, these strategies illuminate the path through sleep's challenges, guiding the weary traveler to the vital embrace of night's tranquility.

In this exploration of nighttime routines and the sanctity of sleep, we discover a series of actions and a philosophy of evening repose, a reverence for the night's role in our well-being. It is a practice that honors the complexity of sleep's influence on our lives, acknowledging its sacred place in the cycle of our existence. Through the deliberate crafting of routines, environments, and strategies to overcome sleep's obstacles, we weave a nightly tapestry of restoration, each thread a silent testament to our commitment to health, balance, and the profound renewal that unfolds in the embrace of sleep.

Reflective Journaling for Inner Peace

In the quiet spaces between our actions and thoughts, reflective journaling unfurls like a ribbon, connecting our present selves with the essence of our experiences and emotions. This practice, often overlooked amidst more tangible self-care activities, can illuminate the caverns of our inner world, shedding light on the contours of our joys, fears, and aspirations. At its core, reflective journaling is an act of dialogue with the self, mapping the landscape of our psyche with words as our guides. Through this exploration, we uncover patterns in our thoughts and behaviors, revealing the undercurrents that steer our emotional well-being. While sometimes uncomfortable, this revelation paves the way for stress relief, allowing us to confront and navigate the complexities of our emotions with clarity and compassion. Moreover, translating thoughts into written words engages the brain in problem-solving, often leading to insights and resolutions that remain elusive in mental rumination.

Embarking on the journey of reflective journaling begins

with the most straightforward steps: selecting a notebook and a pen that feel like extensions of oneself, tools that invite confession and exploration. This initial choice sets the tone for the practice, imbuing it with a sense of ritual and intention. Consistency in journaling, while beneficial, should not become a source of pressure; instead, it is the regular return to this practice, whether daily or weekly, that weaves it into the fabric of our lives. Overcoming blocks to journaling—be it the fear of confronting uncomfortable truths or the belief that one's thoughts are too mundane—requires patience and the understanding that there is no 'wrong' way to journal. Every entry, regardless of its coherence or depth, is a step towards self-discovery and peace.

To aid in the excavation of the self, journal prompts serve as lanterns, illuminating paths through the often tangled forest of our inner lives. "What moment today was I most grateful for and why?" invites a reflection on the day's gifts, fostering an attitude of gratitude. "When did I feel most at peace today, and what was I doing?" helps identify sources of tranquility in our daily lives. For deeper exploration, prompts such as "What fear is holding me back from pursuing my dreams?" or "How does my reflection in the mirror differ from how I see myself on the inside?" challenge us to confront and articulate the complexities of our self-perception and aspirations. These prompts, varied and probing, encourage a journey into the self that is as broad as it is deep, covering the expanse of our experiences, emotions, and dreams.

Transforming journaling into a ritual magnifies its benefits, elevating it from a mere activity to a cornerstone of one's self-care practice. This ritualization involves setting aside a specific time and place for journaling, accompanied by the gentle flicker of a candle or the soothing strains of instrumental music. In this sacred space, journaling becomes a meditative act, a time set apart from the rush of life for introspection and calm. In these moments of quiet communion with the self, journaling transcends the act of writing, becoming a conduit for inner peace. Through the rhythmic dance of pen on paper, we lay bare the contents of our hearts and minds, engaging in a process of self-discovery that brings clarity to our thoughts, relief to our stresses, and solutions to our problems.

In the grand tapestry of self-care, reflective journaling stands out as a thread of introspection and insight, weaving through the fabric of our daily lives to strengthen our relationship with ourselves. It teaches us the art of listening to our inner voice and valuing our experiences and emotions enough to record and reflect upon them. This simple yet profound practice not only aids in stress relief and problem-solving but also fosters a deep, abiding sense of peace within. It reminds us that amidst the chaos of the external world, a sanctuary of calm and understanding resides within, accessible through the pages of a journal.

As we close this chapter on reflective journaling, we understand that the journey to self-discovery and inner peace is personal and perpetual. Each entry in our journal is a step on this path, a testament to our experiences, growth, and resilience. Through writing, we chronicle the narrative of our lives and actively participate in its creation, shaping our story with intention and grace. This practice, interwoven with the other dimensions of self-care explored in this book, forms a holistic approach to well-being that honors the complexity and richness of the human experience.

3

Chapter 3

Transforming Self-Care into a Living Practice

In its ceaseless orbit, the moon offers a silent testament to the power of consistency and adaptation. Night after night, it appears, waxing and waning, ever-present yet ever-changing. This celestial dance, marked by gentle shifts and steadfast presence, mirrors the essence of a practice deeply rooted in the fertile ground of self-care. Here, beneath the moon's watchful gaze, we find a blueprint for setting achievable and transformative goals that evolve with us, guiding our steps like the moonlight that turns the tide.

Setting Achievable Self-Care Goals

Realistic Goal Setting

In self-care, setting goals is akin to planting a garden. Each goal holds potential like a seed but requires the right conditions to flourish. The soil of realism, enriched with the awareness of our current capabilities and limitations, provides the foundation.

Watered with commitment, these goals can grow, but without the nourishment of realistic expectations, they risk withering under the harsh sun of overwhelm. A goal to meditate for an hour daily might tower like an oak in the imagination but may prove more manageable and equally nourishing as a sapling—perhaps starting with five minutes of mindfulness upon waking. This approach ensures that goals enhance our well-being without becoming another hurdle to overcome.

S.M.A.R.T.Goals

The framework of S.M.A.R.T. (Specific, Measurable, Achievable, Relevant, Time-bound) goals introduces a structure to the often nebulous realm of self-care, transforming desires into tangible paths. Imagine deciding to increase water intake—a goal that, while beneficial, lacks clarity. Applying the S.M.A.R.T. approach transforms this aim: "I will drink six glasses of water daily for the next month." Here, specificity and measurability illuminate the path; achievability aligns with current habits, relevance connects to the broader desire for hydration, and time-bound nature offers a frame to assess progress. Such structured goals turn the wheel of self-care forward, moving us closer to our aspirations with each measured step.

Balancing Aspirations with Practicality

The bricks of balance build the bridge between lofty aspirations and daily practicalities. It's recognizing that the pursuit of self-care, while noble, must coexist with the demands of life—a dance between reaching for the stars and keeping feet firmly on the ground. For instance, aspiring to cook nutritious meals at home is commendable. Yet, the practicality of preparing a complex recipe fades on days filled from dawn to dusk. Balance might mean having pre-prepared healthy options or choosing simple, quick-to-prepare dishes that nourish without stress. This equilibrium ensures that self-care goals enrich life rather than add to its burdens.

Adjusting Goals Over Time

Change is the only constant in life—a truth that self-care goals must mirror to remain relevant and supportive. Flexibility in goal setting is not a sign of weakness but a recognition of life's fluid nature. A goal set at the year's start to jog outdoors may clash with the arrival of winter's chill. Instead of clinging rigidly to this goal, adjusting it to include indoor physical activities keeps the spirit of the goal alive while adapting to the present reality. This willingness to mold our goals ensures they continue to serve us, evolving as we do, reflecting our journey's dynamic nature.

Textual Element: Checklist for Setting S.M.A.R.T. Self- Care Goals

1. **Specific**: Define what you want to achieve with as much detail as possible.

• Instead of "exercise more," specify "walk 30 minutes after dinner."

2. **Measurable**: Ensure you can track your progress.

• Mark days on a calendar when you complete your walk.

3. **Achievable**: Set goals within your reach, considering your current lifestyle.

• If evenings are hectic, a morning walk might be more doable.

4. **Relevant**: Align your goals with your broader well-being aspirations.

• Choose activities you enjoy; if walking isn't appealing, perhaps dancing or yoga.

5. **Time-bound**: Give yourself a deadline to work towards.

• Aim to establish this habit over the next two months.

In setting consistent yet adaptable goals that follow the moon's lesson, we cultivate a self-care practice that grows with us, shedding light on our path and guiding us through the night.

Tracking Your Self-Care Journey: Tools and Apps

Benefits of Tracking

In the intricate weave of self-care, the threads of awareness and accountability hold a distinct tension, drawing the fabric taut and lending it both form and function. To track one's self-care activities is to cast a light on the shadowed paths of our routines, illuminating the patterns that foster growth and those that hinder it. This illumination, stark in its honesty, offers a mirror to our habits, reflecting the reality of our commitments to ourselves. The act of recording not only serves as a tangible testament to our endeavors but also fortifies our resolve, transforming ephemeral intentions into concrete actions. Through this lens of accountability, the value of tracking becomes apparent, transforming the nebulous concept of self-care into a quantifiable entity that can be measured, assessed, and, most critically, improved.

Recommended Tools and Apps

In the digital age, the tools to track our self-care journey evolve with the same rapidity that characterizes our lives. From applications that chart our water intake and sleep patterns to platforms that encourage mindfulness and physical activity, the array of options caters to a broad spectrum of needs and preferences. Consider, for instance, apps designed to monitor hydration—simple yet effective in reminding us to nourish our bodies with the essence of vitality: water. Or the sleep trackers that analyze the quality of our rest, offering insights into the patterns that disrupt our slumber and suggestions to enhance it. For those seeking the calm in the storm of daily life, mindfulness apps provide guided meditations, breathing exercises, and moments of reflection, all at our fingertips. Physical activity, too, finds its digital counterpart in apps that log workouts, track progress, and even offer virtual companionship in the form of community challenges. These digital tools, each serving a unique facet of self-care, collectively provide a comprehensive approach to monitoring and enhancing our well-being.

Analog vs. Digital Tracking

Yet, for all the convenience and sophistication of digital trackers, the analog methods—journaling, planners, bullet journals—hold their ground, offering a tactile, profoundly personal approach to tracking self-care. The act of writing, the pen gliding across the paper, provides a moment of pause, a meditative break from the screen-laden landscape of our lives. This method, rooted in tradition, allows for customization that mirrors the unique contours of our self-care journey, free from the constraints of predetermined categories and metrics. Here, in the pages of a journal or planner, the narrative of self-care unfolds in handwritten notes, sketches, and reflections, a story told in ink and intention. The choice between digital and analog tracking does not hinge on the superiority of one over the other but on the alignment with individual preferences, lifestyles, and goals. Each method, with its distinct advantages, supports the practice of self-care, reinforcing the habits that lead to well-being.

Reflecting on Progress

The culmination of tracking, whether through bytes or ink, lies in the act of reflection, a deliberate pause to sift through the accumulated data of our self-care practices. This reflection, far from a cursory glance, demands a deep engagement with our actions and their outcomes, a willingness to question and to learn. It asks us to celebrate the milestones reached, acknowledge the setbacks encountered, and discern the patterns that emerge from the tapestry of our efforts. In this reflective process, progress is measured not just in achieving goals but in the insights gained, the habits formed, and the resilience built. Here, in the quiet contemplation of our journey, the actual value of tracking reveals itself, offering a road map of where we've been, where we stand, and, most importantly, where we wish to go. Through this lens, each entry and each data point becomes a beacon, guiding our steps on the ever-evolving path of self-care.

Cultivating Self-Compassion and Forgiveness

In the quiet introspection that self-care demands, the cultivation of self-compassion and forgiveness emerges as a profound act of kindness towards oneself—a nurturing that allows for growth and healing in the garden of the soul. This practice, woven into the fabric of self-care, acknowledges the human condition's inherent imperfection and the inevitable stumbles on the path to wellness. It is an acceptance that, despite best efforts, setbacks are not markers of failure but milestones of learning and growth. Herein lies the essence of self-compassion: the gentle embrace of one's experiences with a heart open to forgiveness and understanding.

Understanding Self-Compassion

At its core, self-compassion is the ability to hold oneself in a space of understanding and kindness, especially during problematic or perceived inadequacy. It is a turning inward with empathy, recognizing that suffering and personal shortcomings are part of the shared human experience. This compassionate self-acknowledgment shifts the narrative from isolation and self-reproach to shared humanity and self-empathy. The role of self-compassion in effective self-care is profound, acting as a salve to the soul, soothing the wounds of self-criticism, and fostering an environment where healing and growth can flourish.

Practices for Self-Compassion

Cultivating self-compassion flourishes through practice, with mindful self-compassion (M.S.C.) exercises and affirmations as tools for fostering this nurturing mindset. M.S.C. practices, rooted in the mindfulness tradition, encourage a balanced awareness of one's emotions, observing them without judgment and with an open heart. One such practice involves the "Self-Compassion Break," where, in moments of distress, one pauses to acknowledge the pain ("This is tough"), remind oneself of the shared human experience ("Others feel this way too"), and offer self-kindness ("May I be kind to myself"). Alongside, affirmations—positive, compassionate statements directed towards oneself—reinforce this self-compassion. Phrases such as "I am enough," "I forgive myself for my mistakes," and "I am worthy of kindness" serve as gentle reminders of one's intrinsic value and deservingness of compassion.

The Role of Forgiveness

Integral to the tapestry of self-compassion is the thread of forgiveness, particularly in self-directed forgiveness. This aspect acknowledges that missteps are inevitable in pursuing self-care or personal goals. Forgiving oneself for these perceived failures or setbacks liberates one from the chains of self-blame and regret, paving the way for emotional well-being. Self-forgiveness is acknowledging one's humanity—an understanding that mistakes are not a reflection of one's worth but stepping stones to growth. When woven into the daily practice of self-care, this forgiveness becomes transformative, allowing individuals to move forward with a lighter heart and a clearer mind, unburdened by the weight of past grievances against themselves.

Overcoming Self-Criticism

The shadow that often looms large on the path of self-care is self-criticism—a harsh internal dialogue that undermines one's efforts and worth. Overcoming this self-criticism requires a conscious shift towards a more compassionate and forgiving inner dialogue. Strategies for this transformation include "thought replacement," where critical thoughts are acknowledged and then consciously replaced with kinder, more compassionate reflections. Additionally, the "best friend" technique, where one speaks to oneself as one would to a dear friend, offers a perspective shift, encouraging kinder and more supportive self-talk. By fostering a gentler internal dialogue, these practices enhance one's well-being and strengthen the resolve to continue on the self-care journey with kindness and understanding.

In the cultivation of self-compassion and forgiveness, the landscape of self-care is enriched, offering a foundation built not on self-criticism and unrealistic expectations but on kindness, understanding, and forgiveness. This approach, marked by a gentle acknowledgment of one's humanity and inherent worth, fosters a nurturing environment conducive to growth, healing, and a more profound sense of peace. Through consistent practice and mindful reflection, the seeds of self-compassion and forgiveness blossom into a resilient and loving relationship with oneself, illuminating the path of self-care with the light of empathy and understanding.

Overcoming Self-Care Plateaus

In the undulating landscape of self-care, plateaus emerge as natural topographies, spaces where the vigor of ascent levels into expanses of uniformity. These plateaus, marked by stagnation in practices or a waning of motivation, whisper of a need for renewal, for shifts in the patterns that once propelled forward momentum but now tether the spirit in sameness. Recognizing these plateaus necessitates a keen observation of one's internal rhythms, an attunement to the subtle cues of disinterest or mechanical adherence to routines once vibrant with intention. In acknowledging these plateaus, the opportunity for growth unfurls a chance to breathe new life into the practices that compose the mosaic of self-care.

In the quest to breathe vitality into routines grown stale, innovation becomes the compass guiding us through the terrain of sameness. This innovation might manifest in the infusion of variety into physical activities, replacing the monotony of solitary exercises with the dynamic energy of group classes or the fresh challenge of a new sport. Similarly, the realm of mental and emotional care invites a reimagining of practices, perhaps through exploring varied meditation techniques or incorporating creative outlets like painting or journaling, which bring color to the palette of self-care. This refreshment of routines serves not merely to overcome the plateau but to elevate the practice of self-care into a dynamic engagement with oneself, a dialogue that is ever-evolving and rich with discovery.

The quest for inspiration is a beacon, guiding us beyond the familiarity of well-trodden paths to the fresh terrain of novel ideas and perspectives. This inspiration might be sought in the wisdom of books that explore the philosophies of wellness and self-growth, offering new frameworks for understanding and engaging with self-care. Communities, whether in the warmth of local gatherings or the expansive networks of online platforms, provide fertile ground for exchanging ideas, experiences, and support, illuminating the multitude of ways self-care can be interpreted and enacted. Experts in various domains of wellness offer yet another wellspring of inspiration, their insights and practices providing fresh perspectives that challenge and enrich our understanding of self-care. In embracing these sources of inspiration, motivation finds renewal, kindled by the sparks of new knowledge and the resonance of shared experiences.

The fluid nature of life, with its seasons of change and growth, calls for an adaptation in our self-care goals and practices. This flexibility allows for the evolution of our engagement with self-care in alignment with our shifting needs and circumstances. This adaptation might manifest in recalibrating physical goals, recognizing the body's changing needs and capacities, or refining mental and emotional practices to address the nuances of evolving challenges and aspirations. It underscores the importance of holding self-care goals with open hands, ready to mold and adjust them in response to the whisperings of our inner selves and the changing landscapes of our lives. By remaining open to this evolution, self-care remains a relevant and responsive companion on our journey, reflective of our growth and supportive of our well-being.

In navigating the plateaus of self-care, the journey unfolds with a recognition of the need for renewal, an innovation in practices, an inspiration drawn from the wellsprings of knowledge and community, and an adaptation of goals to the rhythms of change. These steps, taken with intention and openness, guide us beyond the stretches of sameness, renewing our engagement with the practices that nurture our bodies, minds, and spirits. Through this continued engagement, self-care transcends the realm of routine, becoming a vibrant and evolving dialogue with ourselves, rich with the potential for discovery and growth.

The Role of Personal Accountability

In the intricate dance of self-care, personal accountability is the rhythm that keeps each step intentional and grounded in purpose. This silent pact with oneself—to honor the commit- ments made for better health and peace of mind—requires a foundation built on mechanisms of accountability, clear intentions, and the celebration of both effort and consistency. In this realm, self-care transforms from fleeting attempts into a sustained melody of wellness.

Accountability Mechanisms

Navigating the waters of self-care with a compass of accountability involves employing mechanisms that serve as reminders and motivators. Self-check-ins, for instance, offer reflective pauses, moments taken to assess progress and realign actions with goals. These can be nightly reflections or weekly reviews when achievements are acknowledged and deviations addressed. Conversely, accountability partners provide an external source of support and encouragement. Choosing someone—be it a friend, family member, or mentor—who understands and shares your journey toward wellness can amplify your resolve, turning the solitary path of self-care into a shared voyage of discovery and growth. Whether through gentle encouragement or the simple act of sharing goals, accountability partners magnify our commitment, making the journey less daunting and more attainable.

Setting Intentions

The setting of intentions plants the seeds of commitment in the fertile ground of self-care. These intentions, clear and resonant, act as guiding stars in the vast sky of possibilities. They transcend mere goals by embodying the why behind each action, imbuing daily practices with purpose and meaning. For instance, the intention to nurture one's body with nutritious food and regular movement goes beyond losing weight; it speaks to a more profound desire for vitality and longevity, aligning each choice with this intention to feel significant and rewarding. This clarity of purpose fortifies the resolve, turning intentions into actions that weave the fabric of a fulfilling self-care routine.

Celebrating Consistency

In the journey of self-care, the milestones of progress are often subtle, manifesting not in grand achievements but in the quiet consistency of effort. Recognizing and celebrating this consistency becomes an act of affirmation, a way of honoring the commitment to oneself. It acknowledges that the power of self-care lies not in sporadic acts of wellness but in the steady accumulation of small, daily practices. Celebrating this consistency can be as simple as reflecting on completing a week's meditation sessions or marking the end of a month filled with mindful eating. These celebrations, though modest, serve as reminders of the strength found in persistence, reinforcing the value of each step taken on the path of self-care.

Overcoming Obstacles to Accountability

Yet, the path of accountability has challenges and obstacles that can cloud intentions and dampen resolve. Procrastination, forgetfulness, and the lack of immediate results often emerge as barriers, casting shadows of doubt and discouragement. Over- coming these obstacles requires strategies that address both the root causes and their manifestations. For procrastination, breaking down goals into smaller, more manageable tasks can reduce the overwhelm that stalls action. For forgetfulness, setting reminders—through apps or simple sticky notes—can serve as beacons, guiding back to the path of self-care. And in facing the slow unveiling of results, cultivating patience becomes critical, a reminder that self-care is a process, its benefits unfolding in the gentle progression of time, not the abrupt revelation of change. Through these strategies, the obstacles that once seemed impossible become stepping stones, each an opportunity to strengthen the resolve and deepen the commitment to personal accountability in self-care.

This exploration of personal accountability within self-care intertwines accountability mechanisms, setting clear intentions, celebrating consistency, and strategies for overcoming obstacles, forming a robust framework for sustaining self-care practices. By acknowledging these facets and integrating them into the daily rhythm of life, self-care evolves from sporadic attempts into a harmonious and enduring melody of wellness.

Integrating Self-Care Into Family Life

Family Self-Care Plans

In the intricate weave of familial bonds, the integration of self-care emerges as an essential thread, reinforcing the fabric of family life with resilience and harmony. Crafting a family self-care plan demands a delicate balance, a dance of individual needs and collective rhythms. This orchestration begins with a communal gathering where each voice can articulate its needs, desires, and visions of well-being. From the youngest to the eldest, every member contributes, painting a mosaic of self-care that reflects the diversity within the unity of the family. Such plans include shared activities that nurture the body and spirit, from weekend nature hikes that breathe fresh air into routines to evening storytelling that weaves tales of wonder and wisdom. Equally, these plans respect the sanctity of individual self-care practices, ensuring each member has the time and space to pursue personal rejuvenation rituals. Through this collective endeavor, families can create a tapestry of care that supports each member while fostering a deepened sense of connection and understanding.

Modeling Self-Care for Children

In parenthood, actions speak with the clarity of a bell, resonating through the corridors of a child's perception, molding beliefs and behaviors with silent potency. Modeling self-care behaviors for children thus becomes a paramount duty, a gift of knowledge passed through the living example of one's practices. With their keen eyes and open hearts, children absorb the nuances of self-care observed in their guardians—be it the tranquility found in a parent's meditation, the joy in a caregiver's dance, or the discipline of a grandparent's morning walk. These observed rituals become the lexicon of well-being for the young, teaching them the language of self-care through the syntax of daily life. Incorporating self-care into family routines serves the individual and becomes a legacy of health passed down, a heritage of habits that nourish and sustain across generations.

Self-Care for Caregivers

Amidst the giving, the constant outpouring of care and attention, caregivers often find themselves adrift in the sea of their duties, their own needs fading like footprints on a beach, washed away by the tides of responsibility. Yet, the essence of providing care springs from the well of one's well- being, a truth that underscores the importance of caregivers embracing self-care with the same enthusiasm with which they attend to others. Strategies for integrating self-care into the life of a caregiver include allocating specific times dedicated to self-nurturance, be it through the solace found in reading or the vitality sparked by exercise. Equally vital is cultivating a support network, a circle of understanding and assistance that can share the weight of caregiving responsibilities, offering respite and relief. Through these practices, caregivers can maintain their reservoir of energy and compassion, ensuring that the care they give is sustained by the care they receive.

Family Communication

At the heart of integrating self-care into family life pulses a vital component—communication. This dialogue, open and continuous, serves as the bridge over which understanding and support can flow freely among family members. It involves not only articulating one's own needs and boundaries but also receptive listening to the needs and boundaries of others. Such communication fosters an environment where self-care is not seen as a solitary act but as a communal value, respected and upheld by all. It encourages negotiating time and resources, ensuring that each member's self-care practices are supported and facilitated. Through open communication, families can navigate the complexities of individual and collective needs, crafting a shared life that honors and reflects the importance of caring for oneself and each other.

In the domain of family life, weaving self-care into the fabric of daily existence becomes an act of love, a testament to the understanding that well-being is both a personal journey and a collective voyage. The practice of self-care transforms through the thoughtful creation of family self-care plans, the powerful modeling of self-care behaviors for children, the attentive self-care of caregivers, and the open channels of family communication. It becomes not just an individual endeavor but a shared commitment, a chorus of care that sings of unity, understanding, and the deep, abiding love that binds families together.

Self-Care in Times of Transition and Change

In the ebb and flow of existence, transitions stand as thresholds, gateways between what was and is yet to unfold. These periods of change, be they as monumental as a seismic shift in career paths or as subtle yet profound as the evolution of family dynamics, beckon for navigation rooted in self-care. The essence of maintaining self-care practices during these transformative phases lies in preserving routines and acknowledging and embracing change as an integral component of growth. Within this embrace, strategies for sustaining self-care practices reveal themselves, offering stability amidst the flux of transition.

Navigating life's transitions with self-care as a compass involves an acute awareness of our internal and external landscapes. This awareness acts as a guide, illuminating the path through uncharted territories of change. Key to this navigation is the prioritization of practices that ground and center, whether through the meditative calm of mindfulness exercises or the physical anchoring provided by regular exercise. However, the real challenge and opportunity lie in the fluidity of adaptation, in understanding that self-care routines established in past seasons may require recalibration to align with new circumstances. This recalibration is a delicate act that demands honesty in acknowledging the shifts in our needs and creativity in adapting practices to meet these evolving demands. Adapting self-care routines to fit new circumstances and challenges begins with accepting change as an inevitable and enriching aspect of life. This acceptance paves the way for re-evaluating self-care practices, inviting innovation and flexibility. For instance, a move to a new city might transform solitary morning jogs into exploratory walks through unknown streets, turning exercise into an adventure. Similarly, a shift in career paths might necessitate finding pockets of peace in a busier schedule, perhaps through shorter, more focused periods of meditation or by integrating mindfulness into daily tasks. The key lies in the willingness to mold self-care practices to fit the contours of our evolving lives, ensuring that these practices remain relevant, supportive, and enriching.

At the heart of navigating transitions is cultivating emotional resilience, a quality that self-care deeply nurtures.

This resilience is the bedrock upon which our ability to weather changes and embrace uncertainty rests. It is fostered through practices that strengthen our emotional and psychological foundations, from the cathartic release in expressive writing to the grounding presence cultivated in mindfulness. Emotional resilience also grows through self-compassion and extending kindness and understanding to oneself during periods of upheaval. This compassionate embrace of our vulnerabilities allows us to move through transitions with grace and grit, viewing these periods not as upheavals but as opportunities for growth and renewal.

Support systems play an indispensable role in bolstering self-care during times of transition. These networks, composed of close family, trusted friends, or supportive communities, provide an external scaffold of encouragement, understanding, and practical assistance. The importance of leaning on these support systems cannot be overstated, for they offer a mirror reflecting our strengths and a safety net catching us in moments of doubt. Seeking out new communities, especially in times of significant change such as relocation or a career shift, can also provide a sense of belonging and continuity. These new connections connect the past to the present and future, ensuring that even amidst change, we are not adrift but anchored in a web of supportive relationships.

In the symphony of life, transitions are inevitable movements, shifts in melody and tempo that bring depth and complexity to the composition. Navigating these transitions with self-care as a guiding principle allows us to move through them with awareness, grace, and resilience. It calls for an adaptation of routines, a cultivation of emotional resilience, and a leaning into support systems, all of which ensure that even in times of change, our commitment to self-care remains unwavering. Through this commitment, we find stability amidst flux and the opportunity to grow, expand our horizons, and embrace the fullness of our evolving lives.

Building a Personalized Self-Care Kit

Navigating the ebbs and flows of daily existence demands not just resilience but tools that anchor us to practices of self- soothing and inspiration. Therefore, a self-care kit emerges as a tangible manifestation of our commitment to well-being, a collection of items meticulously chosen to act as conduits to tranquility, motivation, and joy. This assemblage, unique to each individual, serves as a reminder of the importance of moments stolen from the rush of responsibilities for self- renewal. Within the contents of this kit lies the power to momentarily transcend the mundane, offering a portal to spaces of calm, reflection, and invigoration.

Essentials of a Self-Care Kit

At the heart of each self-care kit is a core of essentials that resonate deeply with our narratives of comfort and rejuvenation. These essentials do not conform to a universal template but reflect our journeys' uniqueness and our needs' diversity. For some, a vial of lavender oil, with its soothing scent, serves as a quick escape to serenity, its aroma a vehicle to a more centered self. For others, a bundle of loose-leaf tea, each sip a warm embrace, becomes a ritual of relaxation and introspection. Including a journal, its blank pages are a canvas for our thoughts, allowing for the unburdening of the mind and transforming swirling thoughts into structured reflections.

Similarly, the soft, tactile comfort of a knitted shawl or the weighted assurance of a stress ball can offer immediate physical anchors to the present, grounding us in the here and now.

Physical vs. Digital Kits

The duality of our existence in both tangible and virtual realms calls for a recognition of the role of both physical and digital self-care kits in our wellness practices. With their tactile nature, physical kits engage our senses directly, offering a hands-on approach to self-care that roots us in the material world. Physically assembling and utilizing this kit becomes a ritual, a deliberate pause in our day dedicated to well-being. Conversely, digital kits, comprised of apps, playlists, and online resources, acknowledge the reality of our digital integration, offering accessible tools with a swipe or a click. These digital collections cater to our need for convenience and immediacy, allowing for a seamless integration of self-care into our digitally mediated lives. The curated playlist that lifts our spirits, the meditation app that guides our breath, and the online journal that stores our reflections all stand as a testament to the adaptability of self-care practices in the digital age.

Ideas and Inspirations

The composition of a self-care kit, be it physical or digital, thrives on personalization, on the infusion of items that speak to our narratives of comfort, inspiration, and joy. For instance, a set of watercolors and a thick pad of paper can offer an outlet for creative expression, a physical manifestation of internal landscapes. A collection of favorite poems or inspirational quotes, whether carried in a pocket or stored on a device, serves as a wellspring of motivation and reflection, a reminder of the resilience and beauty inherent in the human experience. For the auditory soul, a pair of noise-canceling headphones and a carefully curated playlist can transform any space into a sanctuary of sound; each notes a thread in the tapestry of personal harmony. Similarly, a selection of guided imagery recordings can transport the mind to realms of peace and calm, offering respite from the chaos of the external world.

Accessibility and Portability

The actual efficacy of a self-care kit lies not just in its contents but in its accessibility and portability, in its ability to be a constant companion regardless of the fluctuations in our locales and schedules. A compact and thoughtfully assembled physical kit can easily be placed in a day bag or a desk drawer, ensuring that its soothing contents are within reach whenever needed. This portability ensures that our self-care practices are not confined to the home but are woven seamlessly into the fabric of our daily routines, offering solace and rejuvenation on demand. In parallel, digital kits excel in portability, and their presence on our devices guarantees constant accessibility. This omnipresence allows for a fluid integration of self-care practices into our lives, ensuring that, whether we find ourselves in the quiet of our living room or amidst the hustle of a commute, the tools for our well-being are but a touch away, ready to serve us in moments of need.

In crafting a personalized self-care kit, we acknowledge the multifaceted nature of our well-being, recognizing that the journey to self-care is as diverse as personal. Through carefully selecting items that resonate with our narratives of comfort, motivation, and joy, we arm ourselves with tools that not only soothe and inspire but also affirm our commitment to our well-being.

This commitment, encapsulated within the confines of our self-care kits, is a tangible reminder of the importance of nurturing ourselves, offering a beacon of light and warmth in pursuing a balanced, fulfilling existence.

Finding Your Self-Care Community

In the rich tapestry of well-being, the threads interweaving to form a community of like-minded souls stand out in vibrant relief against solitary self-care endeavors. The pursuit of wellness, while deeply personal, gains an enriched dimension when shared, blossoming fully within the fertile soil of collective understanding and mutual support. This communal aspect of self-care, far from diluting the individual journey, amplifies its resonance, creating a chorus of voices that uplifts and sustains each member. The alchemy of shared experience transforms the singular path into a shared pilgrimage, each step buoyed by the knowledge that one does not walk alone.

The benefits derived from immersing oneself in a community that prioritizes self-care are manifold, echoing through the chambers of our physical, emotional, and spiritual well-being. Within these circles, validating one's experiences acts as a balm, soothing the often-isolated journey of personal growth and healing. Validation breeds a sense of belonging, a recognition that one's struggles and triumphs are mirrored in the eyes of another, fostering a profound sense of connection. Moreover, the collective wisdom of a community serves as a rich repository of strategies, insights, and inspirations, a wellspring from which all may draw. The sharing of resources, from practical advice on navigating the challenges of daily self-care to recommendations on tools and practices, enriches the individual's toolkit, broadening the horizon of possibilities.

Engagement with self-care communities, whether they unfold in the warmth of physical gatherings or the expansive realms of digital spaces, requires a mindful approach. When rooted in authenticity and openness, participation nurtures the communal soil, encouraging growth and flourishing. In physical spaces, this may manifest as participation in workshops, group meditations, or shared fitness activities, each interaction woven with the threads of genuine connection and mutual respect. Digital platforms, on the other hand, offer the advantage of transcending geographical limitations and connecting individuals across distances through forums, social media groups, or virtual meet-ups. Here, sharing one's journey, insights, and words of encouragement acts as a digital embrace, bridging the gap between screens and hearts. Contribution to these communities, whether through active participation or the silent support of presence, reinforces the fabric of collective well-being, ensuring its strength and resilience.

The creation and maintenance of safe, inclusive spaces within self-care communities stand as pillars upon which the sanctuary of collective healing rests. In this context, safety extends beyond the physical, encompassing the emotional and psychological realms, where vulnerability is honored and diversity is celebrated. Establishing guidelines that respect boundaries encourages open dialogue, ensures confidentiality, and fosters an environment where individuals feel seen, heard, and valued. Inclusivity, the intentional embrace of diversity in all forms, enriches the community, offering a kaleidoscope of perspectives, experiences, and wisdom. This commitment to safety and inclusivity nurtures trust and openness and serves as a beacon, drawing others to the warmth of understanding and acceptance.

Shared learning and growth, the fruits of communal engagement, blossom in the fertile ground of collective self-care endeavors. When shared, the journey of personal development transforms into a mosaic of collective evolution, each piece a story of individual progress that, when combined, reveals a larger narrative of communal upliftment. Workshops that explore new self-care modalities, group discussions that unpack the layers of well-being, and collaborative projects that aim to extend the reach of self-care practices beyond the confines of the community all contribute to this shared growth. This cooperative learning environment, supported by the mutual exchange of knowledge and experiences, fosters individual and communal transformation. In this shared space of growth and inspiration, the true potential of a self-care community is realized not as a mere gathering of individuals but as a collective force for positive change, both within and beyond its boundaries.

In self-care, discovering or creating a community that mirrors one's values and aspirations is a powerful catalyst for transformation. It offers a space where the journey of well-being is not a solitary trek but a shared voyage, rich with the possibilities of connection, learning, and mutual support. Through engagement with these communities, creating safe and inclusive spaces, and embracing shared growth, the concept of self-care expands, transcending the individual to encompass the collective. Within these communal bonds, the essence of self-care finds its fullest expression, not merely as an act of personal wellness but as a communal celebration of collective thriving.

Embracing Solitude Without Loneliness

In the quiet interludes of our lives, solitude stands as a sanctuary, a realm apart from the clamor of communal existence where the self can commune in silence with the echoes of its thoughts and desires. Though subtle, this distinction between solitude and loneliness is profound, marking the difference between a chosen retreat into the self for rejuvenation and an imposed isolation that echoes with the pangs of disconnection. In its purest form, Solitude enriches the tapestry of self-care, offering a canvas upon which the nuances of our inner landscape can be explored and appreciated without the distraction of external voices. In these moments of deliberate withdrawal, we encounter the richness of our own company, discovering the depths of our thoughts, the resilience of our spirit, and the contours of our creativity.

Activities that flourish in the garden of solitude vary as widely as the individuals who seek them, each chosen pursuit a thread that weaves through the fabric of self-discovery and inner peace. For some, walking alone under the vast expanse of the sky offers a moving meditation, each step a deliberate tread on the path to clarity and calm. The rhythmic cadence of footsteps becomes a mantra, aligning the wanderer with the heartbeat of the world around them, dissolving barriers between the self and the universe. Others may find solace in the silent dialogue of writing, where thoughts that churn in tumultuous silence find a voice on the page, crafting clarity from confusion and understanding from uncertainty. This solitary communion with the written word acts as a mirror, reflecting the complexities of the self back in lines of ink, allowing for a deeper engagement with the intricacies of our being.

Yet, for some, solitude evokes not peace but trepidation, a fear that the whispers of self-doubt and the specters of isolation will rise in the silence. Overcoming this fear demands a gentle approach, a gradual acclimation to the stillness and the space it offers. It begins with the recognition that solitude is not an absence but a presence, not a void but a vessel filled with the potential for introspection and creativity. Small acts of solitary time, carved from the day with intention, can serve as bridges, leading slowly from trepidation to comfort. A few moments spent with a cup of tea, gazing out a window, or a brief walk in a quiet park can introduce the enriching experience of solitude, easing the transition from fear to acceptance.

Balancing the nourishing quiet of solitude with the vibrant tapestry of social interaction is akin to the dance of light and shadow, each element defining and enriching the other. The human spirit, complex and multifaceted, craves both the reflective depth of alone time and the dynamic spark of connection. Finding this equilibrium demands attentive listening to the needs of the self, an awareness of when the soul seeks the serenity of solitude for replenishment, and when it reaches for the warmth of companionship. Social activities, chosen with mindfulness, complement the self-care journey, offering opportunities for laughter, empathy, and shared experiences, illuminating self-discovery in solitude. When mindfully choreographed, this dance between solitude and interaction creates a rhythm of self-care that nourishes all levels, embracing the full spectrum of human experience.

In embracing solitude, we discover not the shadow of loneliness but the light of self-awareness and peace. It is a choice, a deliberate stepping away from the external to engage with the internal, an exploration of the self that enriches and informs our engagement with the world. Through activities that foster self- discovery, strategies that ease the apprehension of solitude, and the mindful balance between alone time and social interaction, solitude is a cornerstone of self-care, a sanctuary within which the self can flourish, unfettered and serene.

Revisiting and Revising Your Self-Care Plan

In the ballet of existence, self-care choreographing movements are both subtle and grand, requiring us to make the initial gesture of commitment and re-evaluate its form and rhythm continually. The dynamic nature of self-care, much like the ebb and flow of the tides, calls for a vigilant reassessment and recalibration, ensuring that what we practice in the name of wellness aligns with our present needs and circumstances. It is an acknowledgment that the self is not a static entity but a constellation of evolving desires, challenges, and insights, each demanding flexibility in our approach to care. This evolution, far from a sign of previous missteps, signals growth, a deepening understanding of the self that necessitates adapting practices once held dear.

In the labyrinth of daily life, where routines establish comfort and predictability, the prospect of revising one's self-care plan might seem daunting, a venture into unknown terrains that promises as much uncertainty as it does potential for renewal. Yet, within this process lies the key to a more authentic, reflective practice of self-care that mirrors our lives' current landscape with fidelity. To navigate this process, a structured approach unwinds before us, inviting introspection and action in equal measure. It begins with the simple yet profound act of questioning, an inquiry into the heart of our self-care practices. Questions such as, "Does this activity still bring me peace, or has it become another task to check off?" or "What new challenges or desires have emerged since I last evaluated my self-care routine?" serve as lanterns, illuminating the aspects of our practice ripe for revision.

This questioning unfolds in the quiet moments we carve for reflection, a sacred pause in the whirlwind of existence where we can turn inward and listen. Here, in the embrace of solitude, insights surface, whispering of needs unmet and aspirations yet to be pursued. Armed with these revelations, we stand ready to weave them into the fabric of our self-care plan, infusing old practices with new life or introducing entirely new rituals that resonate with our current selves. Incorporating insights into our self-care regimen is less about discarding what no longer serves and more about adapting and expanding, ensuring our practices are as multifaceted and vibrant as we are.

Yet, even when it promises growth, change often carries a shadow of reluctance, a hesitance to step away from the familiar. Embracing change in our self-care practices demands recognizing its necessity and celebrating its potential to deepen our relationship with ourselves. It is a leap of faith, a trust in our capacity to adapt and flourish amidst new care configurations. This embrace is not a renunciation of past practices but an acknowledgment of their role in our journey, a foundation upon which newer, more relevant practices can be built. It is a dance of gratitude and anticipation, honoring where we have been while looking forward to where we are going.

Documenting these shifts in our self-care practices serves as a map and a memoir, a record of where we have journeyed in the wellness landscape. A self-care journal or log becomes the repository of this evolution, pages that bear witness to the fluctuations of our needs and the adaptability of our care. In these records, we trace the arc of our growth, noting the practices that have served their purpose and those newly adopted rituals that light our way. This documentation, far from a mere record, becomes a mirror, reflecting the depth of our commitment to self-care and the breadth of our journey. It is a testament to our resilience, a chronicle of change that celebrates our ability to navigate the shifting sands of existence with grace and intention.

In continually revisiting and revising our self-care plan, we engage in an intimate dialogue with the self. This conversation acknowledges the fluidity of our needs and the constancy of our commitment to wellness. This process, iterative and reflective, ensures that our self-care practices remain a true reflection of who we are at any given moment, a tapestry of care that evolves with us, echoing the richness of our inner landscapes. Through this journey, we affirm the dynamic nature of self-care, embracing the changes that come as markers of growth and adaptability and documenting our path to honor our progress and guide our future steps.

Celebrating Self-Care Milestones and Successes

In the intricate dance of self-care, pausing to acknowledge the milestones met and successes achieved along this path is not merely an act of self-indulgence but a critical component of the journey itself. This celebration serves as a powerful affirmation, a tangible acknowledgment of progress that fuels the spirit for the ongoing quest towards well-being. Recognizing these achievements, whether they are steps toward a larger goal or the goal itself, reinforces the commitment to self-care, embedding it deeper into the fabric of one's life. It transforms the often intangible self-care process into a series of celebrated victories, each a beacon that lights the way forward, illuminating the path with the warmth of accomplishment.

Celebrating self-care milestones opens myriad avenues, each reflective of the personal nature of the journey. Simple acts of acknowledgment, such as marking the completion of a month-long meditation challenge with a unique token— perhaps a new meditation cushion or a book on mindfulness — serve to commemorate the effort and dedication invested. For milestones that herald significant transformation, more substantial celebrations might be in order, such as a retreat that offers an opportunity to deepen the practice in a nurturing environment surrounded by nature's tranquility. Even the act of creating a visual representation of one's journey, a self-care map adorned with markers of milestones met, serves as both a celebration and a reminder of the ground covered and the peaks yet to be scaled. These acts of celebration, tailored to resonate with personal achievements, honor the commitment to self-care and amplify its significance, embedding it as a valued aspect of one's lifestyle.

Reflecting on the self-care journey, with its undulating landscape of challenges surmounted and progress achieved, offers a moment of profound insight. This reflection is not a mere glance in the rearview mirror but a deep, contemplative gaze that seeks to understand the contours of the journey. It recognizes the hurdles navigated with resilience, the moments of faltering met with renewed determination, and the instances of joy that peppered the path. This reflective practice, often facilitated through journaling or meditative contemplation, comprehensively appreciates the journey's depth. It highlights not just the milestones celebrated but the invaluable lessons gleaned, the subtle shifts in perspective, and the profound transformations that unfolded along the way. In this reflection, the self-care journey reveals itself not as a series of isolated actions but as a cohesive narrative of growth, resilience, and self-discovery.

Sharing the successes and milestones of one's self-care journey with a community or even a close circle of confidants magnifies the celebration, transforming it into a collective affirmation of the journey's value. This act of sharing, whether through intimate conversations, social media posts, or community gatherings, extends the vibration of one's achievements into the wider world. It serves as a personal celebration and an inspiration to others, a testament to the transformative power of dedicated self-care. The shared stories of overcoming, moments of breakthrough, and realization become threads in the larger tapestry of communal well-being, encouraging others to embrace their self-care journey with hope and determination. In this shared space, the celebration transcends the individual, becoming a beacon that lights the way for others, illuminating the path of self-care with the shared glow of collective triumphs. In self-care, celebrating milestones and successes is a testament to the journey's worth, a series of markers that chart the course of personal evolution. These celebrations, reflections, and shared stories weave a rich narrative of progress, embedding the practice of self-care deeply into the tapestry of one's life.

They serve as reminders of the journey's significance, not just as a series of actions undertaken for well-being but as a profound engagement with the self, a commitment to growth and transformation that resonates through every facet of existence. As we move forward, let us carry the lessons learned, the joy of the milestones celebrated, and the shared inspiration of our successes, ready to meet the unfolding path of our self-care journey with renewed vigor and deepened commitment.

4

Chapter 4

Navigating the Tapestry of Self-Care and Expectations

In the labyrinth of self-care, the echoes of our own and others' expectations reverberate against the walls, creating a symphony that can either harmonize with or disrupt our practices. This chapter delves into the delicate balance of managing these expectations, akin to walking a tightrope where the slightest misstep can lead to a fall into the chasm of stress and disappointment. Here, we explore strategies to tread this line precisely, ensuring that our self-care regimen remains a source of rejuvenation rather than a cause for additional pressure.

Managing Expectations: Yours and Others

Balancing Personal Expectations

Setting realistic self-care goals is an art that requires a deep understanding of one's current capabilities and resources. It's like planning a garden; one doesn't plant a sequoia in a small backyard expecting it to thrive. Similarly, aiming to meditate for an hour daily without prior experience can lead to frustration. Start small with five minutes of focused breathing, and gradually increase the duration as your comfort with the practice grows. This approach ensures that self-care enhances well-being without becoming an overwhelming task.

Navigating External Pressures

The weight of societal, familial, and peer expectations can often distort our self-care practices, turning them into performances rather than genuine acts of self-nourishment. Imagine trying to read a book in a crowded cafe, the chatter and clinking cups distracting you from the words on the page. Similarly, external pressures can divert the focus from what truly benefits us to what merely appears beneficial to others. It's essential to distinguish between helpful advice and intrusive demands, filtering the cacophony to focus on what aligns with our self-care needs.

Assertive Communication

Communicating our needs and boundaries assertively is like navigating a river; done skillfully, it allows us to steer clear of conflicts and misunderstandings. When others' expectations threaten to infringe upon our self-care time, expressing our needs clearly and without apologizing is crucial. For instance, explaining to a family member, "I value our time together, but I need an hour alone each evening to unwind and reflect," sets a boundary while affirming the importance of the relation- ship. This clarity prevents resentment from rooting, allowing relationships to flourish alongside our self-care practices.

Adjusting Expectations Over Time

Life is in constant flux, a stream that twists and turns, its currents ever-changing. Our self-care practices must be as fluid as the stream, adaptable to the evolving landscape of our lives. Regularly assessing and adjusting our expectations ensures that our self-care regimen remains relevant and nurturing. For example, a career change might necessitate a shift in one's exercise routine from early mornings to evenings. Embracing this flexibility allows us to maintain a consistent self-care practice that supports us through life's seasons.

Textual Element: Checklist for Managing Expectations in Self-Care

• **Identify your Non-Negotiables-** Pinpoint the aspect of your self-care routine that is essential for your well-being.

• **Communicate clearly-** Use"I" statements to express your self-care needs to others.

• **Seek feedback Thoughtfully-** While open to suggestions, filter advice through your needs and goals.

• **Reassess Regularly-** Every month, reflect on your self-care practices and adjust as necessary.

• **Practice Flexibility-** Be willing to modify your routines in response to life changes, maintaining the essence of your self-care practice.

Managing the expectations surrounding our self-care practices is a dance of balance, communication, and adaptability. It requires us to be both firms in our commitment to self-care and flexible in how we implement it, ensuring that we can navigate the demands of life without sacrificing our well-being.

98

In mastering this balance, we uphold our self-care regimen and foster healthier relationships with ourselves and those around us, creating a harmony that resonates throughout our lives.

The Impact of Social Media on Self-Image and Self-Care

In the digital age, the tapestry of our social interactions has been intricately woven with the threads of online presence, culminating in a landscape where the distinction between the self and the avatar becomes blurred. The realm of social media, with its galleries of curated lives, acts as both a mirror and a canvas, reflecting our desires for affirmation while simultaneously allowing us to paint idealized versions of our existence. This potent and pervasive duality has profound implications for self-image and self-care, challenging our perceptions and shaping our practices subtly and significantly.

Social Media and Self-Perception

The corridors of social media are lined with mirrors of distortion, each reflecting an image that, though familiar, is often an embellishment of our reality. This distortion arises not from the technology itself but from our engagement with it— the selective sharing of triumphs while silencing the struggles, the meticulous crafting of posts that shine with success while shadowing the ordinary. This selective visibility fosters a skewed self-perception, where the metrics of likes and shares become the yardsticks of personal value, and the absence of acknowledgment is a source of self-doubt. The impact on self-care is dual-fold: urging, on the one hand, is an unsustainable pursuit of perfection, while on the other, it is nurturing neglect of the authentic self in favor of the avatar.

Cultivating a Healthy Online Presence

Cultivating a digital garden that flourishes with positivity requires deliberate choices and actions, akin to pruning the overgrowth to let light touch the soil. This cultivation begins with an awareness of the content that feeds our minds and souls—choosing to follow accounts that inspire and uplift while distancing from those that sow seeds of inadequacy or envy. It extends to our contributions to the digital ecosystem, challenging us to share with authenticity and bring forth not just the blooms but also the buds of our lives—acknowledging that beauty resides in growth, striving, and not just achieving. By curating a digital presence that mirrors the multifaceted nature of our lives, we foster an environment where self-care is nurtured through genuine connection and shared humanity.

Digital Self-Care

In navigating the digital landscape, the practice of digital self-care emerges as a beacon, guiding us toward a balanced engagement with technology. This practice encompasses a spectrum of strategies designed to protect and nurture our well-being in the digital realm. Foremost among these is the digital detox, a deliberate withdrawal from digital devices and platforms, allowing the mind and soul to respite from the constant barrage of information and interaction. Whether it spans hours or days, this detox offers a pause, a moment to reconnect with the tactile world, to engage with the self and others in a space unmediated by screens. Additionally, mindful consumption of digital content, an approach that encourages active engagement with our online activities— questioning their impact on our well-being, seeking out content that enriches rather than depletes—becomes a cornerstone of digital self-care, ensuring our online engagements are sources of nourishment rather than neglect.

Real-Life vs. Online Life

The delineation between our online lives and experiences often fades in the glow of digital screens, challenging us to maintain a grounded perspective in the face of curated portrayals. This challenge calls for reclamation of the values found in the unfiltered moments, in the quiet, unshared instances that weave the fabric of our existence. It invites a recognition that the richness of life lies not in the highlight reel but in the behind-the-scenes—the laughter that leaves no trace on a timeline, the tears that fall unseen, the silent victories and whispered losses. By embracing the entirety of our experiences and acknowledging that the actual texture of life is found in its depth rather than its display, we nurture a self-care practice that honors authenticity over appearance and substance over semblance.

In traversing the digital landscape, we find ourselves at the intersection of technology and humanity, where the reflections cast by social media challenge our perceptions and shape our practices. Through deliberate engagement and mindful action, we can navigate this terrain with intention, cultivating an online presence that supports rather than undermines our self-care, embracing practices that protect our well-being in the digital realm, and maintaining a perspective that values the authenticity of our lived experiences. In doing so, we ensure that our journey through the digital age is marked not by the distortion of self but by the celebration of authenticity, fostering a self-care practice that is both grounded and genuine.

Handling Setbacks in Your Self-Care Journey

In the realm where the cultivation of self-care is both a necessity and a privilege, the certainty of encountering setbacks stands as a testament to the human condition's inherent unpredictability. These interruptions, often perceived as barriers to progress, are, in truth, integral to the fabric of personal growth, sewing into our narrative stitches of resilience and adaptability. Acknowledging setbacks not as failures but as inevitable fluctuations in the continuum of care allows for a perspective shift—from viewing them as hindrances to embrac- ing them as opportunities for deepened self-understanding and refinement of practices.

The occurrence of setbacks, far from a rarity, is a commonality shared across the spectrum of individuals committed to self-nurturance. This universality normalizes the experience, stripping it of its power to evoke guilt or self-reproach. Acknowledging this shared experience fosters collective empathy, a reassurance that ebbs and flows are natural components of any endeavor aimed at personal betterment. The foundation for learning from these interruptions is laid within this acknowledgment, a groundwork that transforms obstacles into stepping stones, propelling us forward with renewed insight and vigor.

Strategies for reflecting upon and learning from these interruptions in self-care are manifold, each offering a different lens to examine and extract wisdom from these occurrences. One such strategy involves the practice of reflective journaling, a method that allows for the externalization of thoughts and emotions, providing a tangible form through which to analyze and understand the nature of the setback. This practice encourages a dissection of the event, prompting questions such as, "What external factors contributed to this interruption?" or "How did my response to the event influence its impact on my self-care routine?" Through this reflective inquiry, patterns emerge, clarifying potential vulnerabilities in our self-care regimen and highlighting areas ripe for fortification.

In the face of setbacks, the cultivation of self-compassion emerges as a beacon, guiding us back to a path marked by kindness and understanding. This approach rejects the allure of self-criticism, an easy companion in times of perceived failure, and instead promotes a dialogue with oneself that is nurturing and supportive. Practicing self-compassion involves recognizing the commonality of setbacks and offering oneself the same empathy and encouragement one would extend to a dear friend in similar circumstances. It is a practice that acknowledges our best efforts and forgives our lapses, reinforcing our commitment to self-care not as a rigid regimen but as a fluid, evolving practice that accommodates growth and learning.

The journey back to a consistent self-care routine after a setback is akin to the healing process—gradual, requiring patience and deliberate action. The initial step in this journey involves identifying small, manageable actions that signify a return to self-care. These activities do not overwhelm but instead instill a sense of capability and progress. This might include reintegrating a favored self-care activity into one's daily routine, perhaps beginning with a shortened duration or modified intensity. Additionally, setting micro-goals, quickly attainable achievements that serve as immediate sources of motivation, can reignite the momentum lost during the setback. The essence of bouncing back lies in the incremental reclamation of our self-care practices, which honors our current state while gently nudging us towards re-establishing our routines. In navigating the undulating terrain of self-care, where setbacks emerge as both challenges and teachers, our response to these interruptions defines the resilience and flexibility of our practice. Through the normalization of setbacks, reflective learning, the cultivation of self-compassion, and deliberate steps towards regaining momentum, we transform these experiences from mere interruptions to valuable contributors to our journey of self-care. Within this transformation, our practice deepens, enriched by the understanding and adaptability forged in the crucible of setbacks.

The Connection Between Self-Care and Self-Esteem

Self-esteem, that inner compass guiding our perceptions of worth and capability, flourishes in the fertile ground of consistent self-care practices. This symbiotic relationship, intricate in its weaving, nurtures a self-image that blooms with confidence and resilience. Regular self-care acts as a mirror and map, reflecting our inherent value while guiding us through personal growth and acceptance. In the quiet moments of self-reflection, the deliberate pauses for care, we cultivate a garden where self-esteem can thrive, unshadowed by doubt.

The architecture of our self-esteem is built, in part, through activities that resonate deeply with our core selves, practices that echo our intrinsic worth back to us. Engaging in physical activity, for example, transcends the mere act of movement, transforming into a dialogue of strength and endurance. Each stride, each stretch, whispers of our capabilities, reinforcing a belief in our physical and mental fortitude. Similarly, the pursuit of creative expression—through painting, writing, or any form of art—serves as a conduit for inner exploration, each creation a testament to our unique perspective and talent. This act of making, bringing forth something solely ours, affirms our worth in ways words cannot capture.

Volunteer work, too, plays a pivotal role in this dance of self-care and self-esteem. We encounter our capacity for compassion and impact in extending ourselves to others and touching lives beyond our own. This outward reach, generous in its essence, reflects the significance of our existence within the larger tapestry of humanity. The gratitude and connections forged in giving weave threads of confidence and purpose into our self-image, bolstering our sense of self-worth with the knowledge of our contributions to the world.

Yet, amidst these practices, the specter of negative self-talk often lurks a shadow that dims the light of our self-esteem. This internal critic, relentless in its commentary, carves grooves of doubt and self-deprecation into our minds, undermining the efforts of self-care and eroding our sense of worth. Overcoming this adversary requires a vigilant awareness of our thought patterns and a readiness to intercept and challenge the integrity of these internal narratives. Techniques such as cognitive restructuring come to bear here, offering a method to dismantle these patterns. It involves pausing at the onset of negative self-talk, dissecting the thought for its truth, and rewriting the narrative in a kind and factual manner. Though simple in its description, this practice demands persistence and patience, a commitment to rewire our internal dialogues towards affirmations of strength and worth.

Equally critical in nurturing self-esteem is celebrating personal achievements and acknowledging our efforts and successes, regardless of scale. Often overlooked in pursuing larger goals, this celebration reinforces our sense of accomplishment and capability. It could be as simple as marking the completion of a daily self-care activity with a moment of gratitude or as significant as commemorating a month of consistent self-care practice with a reward that honors the commitment. Each acknowledgment and celebration act as a stepping stone, building a path of confidence and self-assurance. Through these moments of recognition, we affirm that our endeavors matter, our efforts bear fruit, and we are worthy of the care we bestow upon ourselves.

In self-care and self-esteem, the journey is not linear but a spiral, a continuous loop where care nurtures esteem, deepening the commitment to care. This cyclical progression, enriched by activities that affirm our worth, techniques that silence the critic within, and celebrations that honor our achievements, fosters a relationship with ourselves rooted in respect, appreciation, and love. Here, in the fertile ground of self-care, we find the nourishment for our self-esteem to bloom and the strength and resilience to weather the storms of doubt and criticism. In this dance of care and esteem, we discover the true essence of our worth, a realization that shines with the clarity of our inherent value, unmarred by the shadows of insecurity.

Advocating for Your Well-being in Relationships

Within the intricate web of human connections, advocating for one's well-being emerges as a nuanced dance, a delicate interplay of expression and reception that shapes the equality of our interactions and, by extension, the essence of our lives. The ability to articulate one's needs for self-care within the context of relationships is akin to navigating a river whose currents are unpredictable and familiar; it requires a keen understanding of the waters and a confident command of one's vessel. This chapter explores the art of communicating self-care needs, establishing boundaries, maneuvering through the dynamics of resistance, and fostering an environment of mutual support in relationships.

Communicating Needs

The expression of self-care needs is a practice rooted in vulnerability and strength, a paradox that reveals the complexity of our human connections. It demands a clarity of voice and an open heart, inviting those we hold dear into our inner sanctum with trust and honesty. Imagine the delicate unfolding of a flower at dawn, its petals revealing the tender heart within to the light. Similarly, effective communication about our self-care unfolds in layers, each word chosen with care intended to bridge understanding and foster empathy. This dialogue is not a monologue but an invitation to a shared space where needs are not just spoken but heard, where the language of care transcends words to become the very bedrock of the relationship.

Setting and Maintaining Boundaries

Establishing boundaries in relationships is not an act of division but a declaration of respect and self-preservation. It delineates the sacred space in which we operate, marking the parameters within which our well-being flourishes.

Precise and firm, yet permeable to the touchstones of compassion and compromise, these boundaries are the walls of a garden where the self can bloom unimpeded by the overgrowth of external demands. Setting them requires a delicate balance, a gentle yet assertive articulation of where we end and others begin, ensuring that our self-care is not compromised by the needs or expectations of those around us. Maintaining these boundaries is an ongoing endeavor, a vigilant tending to the garden, ensuring that the lines once drawn in the soil of our relationships remain visible and respected, a testament to our commitment to self-preservation and mutual respect.

Navigating Relationship Dynamics

The waters of relationship dynamics are often stirred by resistance and misunderstanding, challenging the steadfastness of our self-care endeavors. Encountering resistance, particularly from those whose opinions we value, can feel akin to navigating a storm; it tests our resolve and demands a steadiness of purpose. The key to maneuvering through these tempests lies not in confrontation but in the art of negotiation, a tactful engagement that seeks to illuminate rather than overshadow. It involves a willingness to explore the roots of resistance, to understand the fears or misconceptions that may lie beneath the surface, and to address them with empathy and insight. This process is not about capitulation but finding a middle ground, a shared territory where all parties acknowledge and respect self-care's importance.

Self-Care and Mutual Support

At its core, the relationship between self-care and mutual support is symbiotic, each nourishing the other in a cycle of growth and understanding.

Cultivating an environment where self-care is not just an individual pursuit but a collective value adds a layer of richness to our interactions, transforming the soil of our relationships into fertile ground for mutual flourishing. This environment thrives on the principles of empathy, where the self-care practices of one are met with encouragement and support by another, creating a network of care that extends beyond the self to encompass the community of connections we cherish. It is a space where caring for oneself becomes a beacon, illuminating the path for others to follow and encouraging a culture of wellness that transcends individual practice to become a shared journey.

In advocating for our well-being within relationships, we engage in profound self-respect and love, a declaration that our needs are valid and worthy of acknowledgment. This advocacy, articulated through clear communication, establishing boundaries, strategic navigation of relationship dynamics, and fostering mutual support, is a testament to our commitment to self-care. It is a commitment to preserving self and enriching all our relationships. It is a recognition that in caring deeply for ourselves, we are better equipped to care for those we hold dear, nurturing resilient connections and imbued with understanding.

Self-Care and Financial Wellness

In the interplay of self-care and financial wellness, an intricate dance unfolds, weaving through the rhythms of daily life with the precision and delicacy of a ballet. Though often overlooked, this dance is pivotal in the grand performance of self-care, for the strains of financial discord can dissonant the most harmonious well-being melodies.

At its core, financial stress acts not merely as a detractor of peace but as a significant barrier to the holistic embrace of self-care, necessitating an approach that melds financial prudence with personal wellness. The link between financial strain and overall well-being is profound, a river whose currents run deep, touching the banks of our lives with the cold spray of reality. The weight of financial unease casts long shadows over our mental and emotional landscapes, clouding our capacity to engage fully with the self-care practices that nourish us. It is within this acknowledgment that financial self-care emerges as a beacon, guiding us towards a shore of stability where the tumultuous waves of worry give way to the calm waters of security. Financial self-care, then, stands not as a separate entity but as an integral component of a holistic self-care plan, a thread in the tapestry that binds our physical, mental, and financial well-being into a cohesive whole.

In this context, budgeting for self-care becomes an act of balancing; economic constraints do not hinder a meticulous arrangement of resources that ensures our capacity for self-nourishment. This balancing act, akin to the careful composition of a meal that satisfies both taste and nutritional needs, requires an awareness of our financial landscape and a prioritization of our well-being expenditures. Practical ways to budget for self-care involve a discerning eye, identifying and allocating funds for activities and practices that yield high dividends in personal wellness. It may include setting aside a modest sum for a monthly massage, recognizing the profound impact of this physical therapy on one's mental state, or dedicating resources to a weekly yoga class that centers and grounds.

The essence of this budgeting lies in its intentionality, the conscious decision to invest in one's well-being, ensuring that financial limitations do not become prohibitive barriers to care.

When viewed through the lens of self-care, financial planning and management transform from mundane tasks to proactive empowerment strategies. This transformation is rooted in the understanding that financial stability contributes significantly to our peace of mind, offering a foundation for the tower of holistic health. Engaging in financial planning is akin to planting a garden for future sustenance; each decision, each allocation of resources, a seed sown for the harvest of long-term well-being. This proactive approach involves managing current resources and anticipating future needs, crafting a financial strategy that accommodates the unforeseen and the expected, and ensuring that our capacity for self-care endures through seasons of plenty and want.

Resources and tools for managing financial wellness abound, offering a plethora of aids designed to weave financial self-care seamlessly into the fabric of our lives. These tools, ranging from budgeting apps that track expenditures with the tap of a screen to financial planning services that offer personalized advice, serve as the instruments through which we orchestrate our financial well-being. Engaging with these resources is akin to learning a new instrument, initially challenging but ultimately rewarding, as the melodies of financial stability harmonize with the rhythms of our daily existence. Online platforms and community workshops provide not just guidance but a space for shared learning, where the experiences of others illuminate our path, offering insights and strategies that enrich our understanding of financial self-care. Through these resources, the daunting becomes manageable, the complex, simplified, and the path to financial wellness, a journey marked by growth, learning, and empowerment. In this exploration of self-care and financial wellness, we traverse the landscape of well-being, acknowledging the profound impact of financial stability on our holistic health. Through the integration of financial self-care into our broader self-care regimen, the crafting of budgets that prioritize our well-being, the adoption of financial planning as a form of proactive self-care, and the utilization of resources and tools designed to enhance our financial wellness, we strengthen the foundation upon which our holistic health rests. In this dance of self-care and financial wellness, we move with grace and intention, each step a testament to our commitment to nurture ourselves fully, embracing the harmony of well-being that resonates through every aspect of our lives.

Addressing Burnout Proactively

Burnout, a shadow that often creeps unnoticed into the corridors of our lives, manifests as a silent thief of joy and motivation, leaving a trail of exhaustion and disillusionment in its wake. Its insidious nature makes early detection vital, a beacon that alerts us to tread carefully on the path we are navigating. The signs of burnout—persistent fatigue, a sense of futility, irritability, and detachment from activities once approached with enthusiasm— serve as the early warnings of a system in distress, signaling the urgent need for intervention.

Self-care practices wield considerable power in the arsenal of tools available to combat the onset of burnout.

These practices, far from mere indulgences, act as bulwarks against the erosion of our well-being. They invite us to pause and indulge in rest and leisure activities that replenish our spent energies, like rain nourishing an arid land, coaxing life into dormant seeds. The act of disconnecting, of stepping away from the continual demands of productivity to bask in moments of stillness or engage in activities purely for the joy they bring, is not an act of defiance against a culture that prizes constant activity but a necessary recalibration of our internal compasses.

Creating a sustainable work-life balance, an endeavor often likened to finding equilibrium on a seesaw, demands a meticulous curation of priorities, an acknowledgment that not all demands carry equal weight. It requires setting boundaries around our time and energy, clearly delineating between work and rest, engagement and withdrawal. This balance does not imply an equal partitioning of hours but a harmony between the demands of our professional lives and our well-being needs. Strategies to achieve this often involve meticulous planning, negotiation of responsibilities, and a willingness to delegate, ensuring that our pursuits outside the sphere of work receive the attention and energy they rightfully deserve.

Yet, there are instances when burnout presses heavily, a burden too challenging to lift with self-care practices alone. In such moments, seeking professional help emerges as a profoundly proactive step, recognizing that the path to recovery sometimes requires the guidance of those trained to navigate these troubled waters. This act of reaching out, far from a concession of defeat, is a testament to our strength, a declaration that our well-being is paramount. Therapists and counselors act as allies, offering strategies to manage stress, techniques to reframe our perspectives, and, importantly, a space where our experiences are validated and understood. In proactively addressing burnout, we engage in a multi-faceted dance. This choreography encompasses early recognition of its signs, the deployment of self-care practices as preventative measures, crafting a life where work and rest coexist in harmony, and the wisdom to seek guidance when the shadows lengthen. This nuanced and layered approach ensures that we remain vigilant guardians of our well-being, capable of navigating the complexities of modern life with resilience and grace.

Nurturing Resilience Through Self-Care

In the intricate dance of existence, resilience emerges not as a static attribute bestowed upon a fortunate few but as a dynamic quality cultivated through self-care. It's within the embrace of life's inevitable ebbs. It flows that the true essence of resilience reveals itself—not as the absence of vulnerability but as the capacity to navigate through adversity with an undiminished spirit. This quality, akin to the enduring nature of a river that carves its path through the landscape despite the rocks and ravines in its way, underscores the profound interplay between self-care and the fortitude to face life's challenges with a steadfast heart.

At the heart of fostering resilience lies the acknowledgment that life, in all its unpredictable glory, presents a spectrum of experiences—each laden with the potential to fortify or fray the fabric of our being. The cultivation of resilience, therefore, becomes an act of conscious engagement with these experiences, an open-hearted willingness to encounter them with a spirit of curiosity and growth. The foundations of resilience are laid in the quiet moments of introspection, the gentle embrace of our inner world, and our deliberate choices in caring for ourselves.

Practices such as mindfulness meditation offer sanctuary, a space where the tumult of the outside world gives way to a tranquil inner landscape. Here, amidst the ebb and flow of breath, we encounter our core, a wellspring of calm and clarity that remains untouched by the chaos that swirls beyond. Similarly, cultivating social connections, those threads that bind us to a community of shared experiences and mutual support serves as a lifeline. These connections remind us of our place within a larger tapestry of human endeavor, offering solace and strength in moments of isolation and doubt.

The perspective with which we approach adversity is pivotal in nurturing resilience. Viewing challenges not as insurmountable obstacles but as opportunities for growth transforms the narrative of our experiences. It shifts the focus from what has been lost to what can be gained, from the pain of the present to the potential for transformation. This reframing is not a dismissal of the hardship but an acknowledgment of its role in the alchemy of personal development. Each encounter with adversity becomes a chapter in the larger story of our resilience, a testament to our ability to rise, time and again, fortified by the lessons learned, and the strength garnered along the way. Resilience is not merely a quality to be called upon in times of crisis but a lifelong practice woven into the fabric of our daily existence through self-care rituals. It demands of us a commitment to continually nurture our well-being and to prioritize practices that replenish our mental, emotional, and physical reserves. This commitment takes shape in the mundane and the extraordinary, in our daily choices to honor our needs, and in the moments of grace we afford ourselves amidst the hustle of life.

We establish that resilience finds its proper expression in the consistency of these practices and the care rhythm. It becomes a melody that plays softly in the background of our lives, a tune that steadies us in the face of turmoil and buoys us in the waters of uncertainty.

The path to resilience, marked by the stones of self-care, is personal and universal, a journey unique to each yet shared by all who navigate the complexities of human existence. It is a path that meanders through landscapes of joy and valleys of despair, illuminated by the light of our inner strength and the support of those who walk with us. By deliberately cultivating practices that ground us, connect us, and reframe our experiences, we build the resilience that sustains us through challenges and enriches our engagement with life. This resilience, nurtured through the embrace of self-care, empowers us to face each new day with a heart undaunted, a spirit unbroken, and a resolve unwavering.

Envisioning Your Future Self: A Self-Care Blueprint

Future-Self Visualization

Imagine standing before a mirror, not one that reflects your current form, but rather, a portal through which you glimpse your future self. This visualization, a practice steeped in the potency of imagination, invites you to conceive of a version of yourself nurtured through dedicated self-care practices. It's akin to planting a garden in your mind where each seed represents a future aspect of your well-being, grown to its fullest potential. Engage deeply with this mental exercise, picturing yourself radiating health, embodying peace, and exuding contentment.

Allow this vision to be detailed; see the vibrancy in your eyes from rested nights, feel the strength in your steps from nourishing movements, and hear the steadiness in your breath from moments of mindfulness. This vivid portrayal serves as an aspiration and a beacon, guiding your choices and practices in the present.

Setting Long-Term Self-Care Goals

With a clear image of your future self as the canvas, setting long-term self-care goals becomes the brush with which you paint the path to this envisioned state. This process transcends mere wishful thinking, grounding your aspirations in actionable, tangible objectives. It's the difference between a nebulous desire for health and a concrete plan to incorporate whole foods into your diet, to meditate daily, or to engage in physical activity that brings you joy. Each goal set is a commitment, a pact made with your future self, acknowledging that the journey to well-being is a marathon, not a sprint. Frame these goals within realistic timelines, understanding that true transformation is gradual and requires patience, persistence, and a gentle acknowledgment of your current starting point.

The Role of Daily Practices

The mosaic of your future well-being is pieced together through the accumulation of daily self-care practices. These bricks pave the road to your envisioned future; each day's efforts are a small but significant step toward your long-term goals. Consider how the ritual of morning hydration prepares your body for the day or how nightly journaling unwinds the mind and cultivates gratitude. Though seemingly modest in isolation, these practices compound over time; their benefits magnify as they become woven into the fabric of your life.

They require a mindful dedication, an everyday choice to prioritize your well-being amidst the myriad demands of life. In these moments, these daily acts of self-care, the foundation for a future enriched with health and happiness is laid.

Adapting and Evolving

As your life's seasons shift, so must your self-care blueprint. This document, a living testament to your commitment to well-being, must remain flexible and open to adjustments as you grow and your circumstances change. Recognize that the strategies and practices that serve you today may need to evolve tomorrow. Embrace this adaptability as a strength that reflects your responsiveness to your body's and mind's changing needs. This willingness to modify your approach ensures that your self-care practice remains relevant and supportive, reflecting your journey toward your envisioned future. It speaks to a deep understanding that self-care is not static but an ever-evolving dialogue with yourself that respects the nuances of your growth and the fluidity of life's constant changes.

As we close this exploration of envisioning your future self and crafting a self-care blueprint, we've traversed the terrain from the potent exercise of future-self visualization to the practicalities of setting long-term goals and embedding daily practices into our lives.

We've acknowledged the necessity of adaptability, embracing the evolution of our self-care strategies as we navigate the shifting landscapes of our lives. This journey, rooted in the present but always with an eye toward the future, is a testament to the transformative power of dedicated self-care. It underscores the understanding that the path to our envisioned future selves is paved with our small, daily choices to serve our well-being. As we move forward, let this blueprint serve as a guide and a living document that reflects our growth, challenges, and victories in pursuing a life enriched by comprehensive self-care.

5

Conclusion

As we draw the curtains on this transformative journey of self-discovery and self-care, we must reflect on the ground we've covered together. From the foundational stones of understanding what self-care truly means to the advanced strategies for weaving it into the very fabric of our lives, this voyage has been one of profound growth and enlightenment. Guided by the 30-day plan, you've seen firsthand the metamorphosis that unfolds when one commits wholeheartedly to nurturing one's well-being.

In today's whirlwind of existence, self-care transcends the realm of luxury to plant its roots firmly in the territory of necessity. The benefits you've reaped—stress alleviation, enriched relationships, or a surge in productivity—are but a glimpse into the vast expanse of rewards that regular self-care practices harbor. Let this be a reminder that caring for oneself is not an act of indulgence but an act of survival and thriving in the modern landscape.

Echoing the core messages of our journey, remember the pillars that uphold the temple of self-care: the beauty of personalization, the wisdom of setting attainable goals, the strength of self-compassion, and the resilience that sustains us through life's ebb and flow. These principles are your compass as you navigate the waters of self-care beyond the initial 30 days, guiding you to shores of continuous discovery and renewal.

Our exploration spanned across the vast terrains of self-care —from the quiet sanctity of morning rituals to the reflective solitude of digital detoxes, from the empowerment of financial wellness to the simple joy of a mindful commute. This diversity in practices underlines the holistic nature of self-care,

a testament to its ability to touch every corner of our lives.

I urge you, dear reader, to view your self-care journey not as a destination but as a perpetual adventure—a path of constant exploration, adaptation, and growth. Stay curious, stay open, and allow yourself the grace to modify your routines as you evolve.

Remember the invaluable role of community and support on this path. Though deeply personal, the journey of self-care need not be solitary. Lean on your network of family, friends, or online comrades to share the weight of challenges and the lightness of successes. Together, we can lift each other to greater heights of well-being. And when the road gets rocky, as it inevitably will, meet your- self with the same kindness and resilience you've cultivated. View every setback as a lesson, every obstacle as an opportunity to deepen your understanding and practice self-care.

So, take that first step if you still need to. Start small with one act of self-care, and let the momentum carry you forward.

The hardest part is often just beginning, but remember—the most extraordinary journeys start with a single step. From me to you, thank you for embarking on this path of self-care with me. I hope the seeds planted throughout these pages blossom into a garden of peace, joy, and fulfillment in your life. I believe in the transformative power of self-care and, more importantly, in you. May you find the strength, courage, and joy in caring for yourself today and always.

SEE THE "REDISCOVERING YOU: A 30 DAY SELF-CARE GUIDE TO MODERN LIVING OFFICIAL WORKBOOK" FOR ADDITIONAL SELF-CARE TIPS, EXERCISES, AND TRACKING SHEETS

SHARING IS CARING!

If you love it, leave a review
and share with your friends!

Scan to leave your book
review

30 Day Self-Care Plan

This 30-day plan incorporates a variety of self-care activities that cater to different aspects of well-being – physical, emotional, mental, and social. Enjoy the journey, adapt the activities to your preferences, and continue practicing self-care beyond the 30 days for ongoing well-being.

Week 1: Mindful Beginnings

Day 1: **Gratitude Journaling**
- Write down three things you're grateful for today.

Day 2: **Morning Meditation**
- Start your day with a 10-minute meditation session.

Day 3: **Nature Connection**
- Spend 20 minutes outdoors, connecting with nature.

Day 4: **Mindful Breathing**
- Practice deep breathing exercises for 5 minutes.

Day 5: **Digital Detox**
- Take a break from screens for at least two hours.

Day 6: **Creative Expression**
- Engage in a creative activity for 30 minutes.

Day 7: **Random Act of Kindness**
- Perform a random act of kindness for someone.

30 Day Self-Care Plan

Week 2: Emotional Wellness

Day 8: **Self-Compassion**
- Write a heartfelt letter of self-compassion.

Day 9: **Mindful Listening**
- Have a mindful conversation with a friend or family member.

Day 10: **Positive Affirmations**
- Create and repeat three positive affirmations.

Day 11: **Music Therapy**
- Listen to your favorite calming music for 20 minutes.

Day 12: **Emotional Check-In**
- Reflect on your emotions without judgment.

Day 13: **Digital Declutter**
- Organize your digital files or emails for clarity.

Day 14: **Body Scan Meditation**
- Practice a body scan meditation for relaxation.

30 Day Self-Care Plan

Week 3: Physical Well-Being

Day 15: **Yoga Session**
- Engage in a 30-minute yoga practice.

Day 16: **Healthy Meal Prep**
- Prepare a nutritious meal from scratch.

Day 17: **Pampering Session**
- Treat yourself to a spa-like self-care day.

Day 18: **Hydration Focus**
- Drink plenty of water throughout the day.

Day 19: **Mindful Eating**
- Eat one meal mindfully, savoring each bite.

Day 20: **Strength Training**
- Engage in 20 minutes of strength-building exercises.

Day 21: **Mindful Movement**
- Take a 20-minute walk or practice your favorite physical activity.

30 Day Self-Care Plan

Week 4: Social Connection

Day 22: **Virtual Social Gathering**
- Arrange a virtual meetup with friends or family.

Day 23: **Acts of Gratitude**
- Write thank-you notes to people who've positively impacted your life.

Day 24: **Reflect on Boundaries**
- Consider and set healthy personal boundaries.

Day 25: **Community Engagement**
- Find a way to contribute to your local community or a cause you care about.

Day 26: **Self-Reflection**
- Journal about your self-care journey and insights.

Day 27: **Mindful Communication**
- Practice mindful communication with someone.

Day 28: **Celebration Day**
- Celebrate your self-care journey with a favorite activity or treat.

Week 5: Growth and Reflection

Day 29: **Set Future Goals**
- Reflect on your self-care journey and set goals for continuing self-care.

Day 30: **Share Your Journey**
- Share your self-care journey with a friend or on social media. Encourage others to embark on their own self-care journeys.

7 Techniques for Stress Management and Inner Peace

1. MEDITATING/PRAYING
2. EXERCISING
3. INTERACTING WITH NATURE
4. DEEP BREATHING
5. VISUALIZALIZING
6. JOURNALING
7. PRACTICING GRATITUDE

3 Exercises for Daily Self-Care

1. Speak positive words of affirmation daily

2. Eat a balanced diet and take a daily vitamin supplement

3. Move your body and get some exercise.

5 Secrets to Boosting Self Esteem

---

1. Set big and small goals. Celebrate ALL achievements!

2. Work in Your Why- Work in a job that allows you to feel purpose and fulfillment.

3. Stop Comparing Yourself...No one is like YOU!

4. Build a support network of close friends and family for when you are feeling down. Remember everyone had bad days.

5. Set boundaries- It's OK to say NO. Pleasing your self is more important than pleasing others.

Journal Prompts

10 Prompts for Journaling and Meditation

What values do you consider most important in life (honesty, justice, altruism, loyalty, etc.)? How do your actions align with those values?

What are your strengths in relationships (kindness, empathy, etc.)?

How does work fulfill you? Does it leave you wanting more?

How do you show compassion to others? How can you extend that same compassion to yourself?

How can you better support and appreciate your loved ones?

What five traits do you value most in potential partners?

What boundaries could you set in your relationships to safeguard your own well-being?

What parts of daily life cause stress, frustration, or sadness? What can you do to change those experiences?

What three changes can you make to live according to your personal values?

Finish this sentence: "My life would be incomplete without ..."

www.ingramcontent.com/pod-product-compliance
Lightning Source LLC
Chambersburg PA
CBHW060238030426
42335CB00014B/1519